101
WAYS TO WORK OUT
ON THE BALL

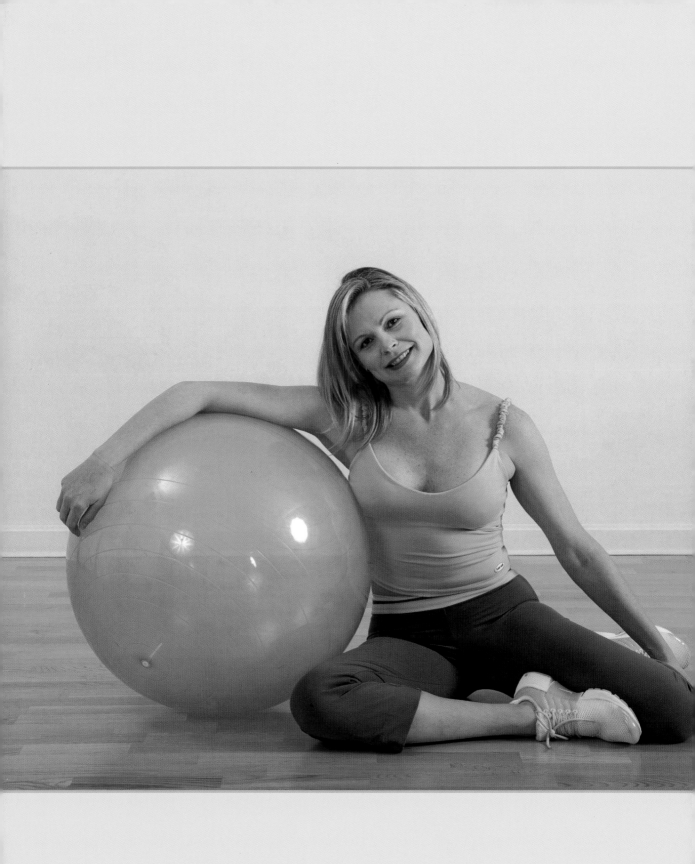

101

WAYS TO WORK OUT ON THE BALL

SCULPT YOUR IDEAL BODY WITH PILATES, YOGA, AND MORE

Elizabeth Gillies

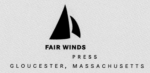

FAIR WINDS
PRESS
GLOUCESTER, MASSACHUSETTS

Text © 2004 by Elizabeth Gillies

First published in the USA in 2004 by
Fair Winds Press
33 Commercial Street
Gloucester, MA 01930

08 07 06 05   4 5

ISBN 1-59233-084-3

Library of Congress Cataloging-in-Publication Data available

Cover and book design by
Laura H. Couallier, Laura Herrmann Design

Printed and bound in Singapore

The information in this book is for educational purposes
only. It is not intended to replace the advice of a physician
or medical practitioner. Please see your health care provider
before beginning any new health program.

For my Dad, Francis D. Gillies, Jr., in loving memory.

His passion for books was truly inspiring.

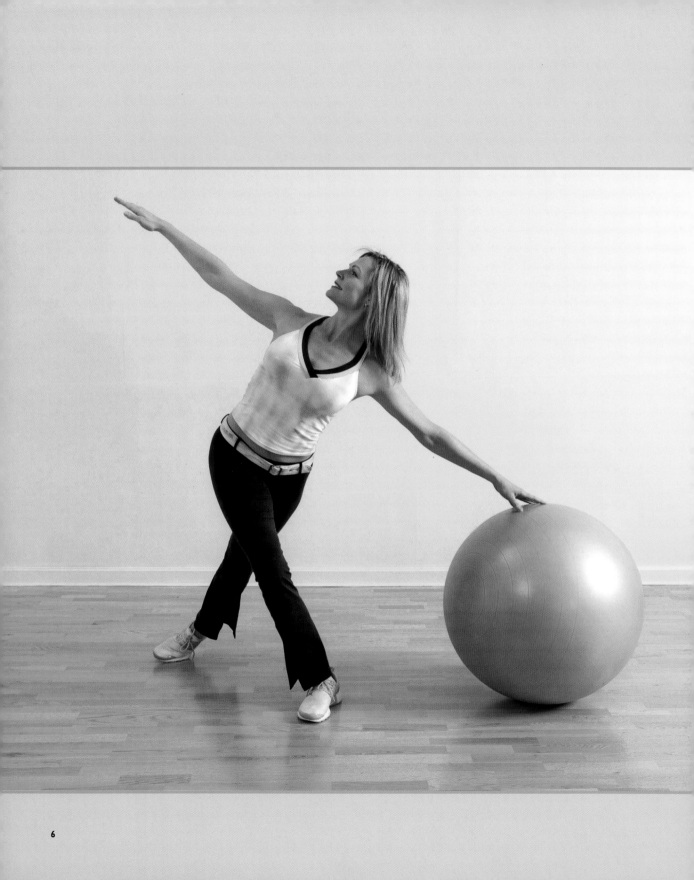

Contents

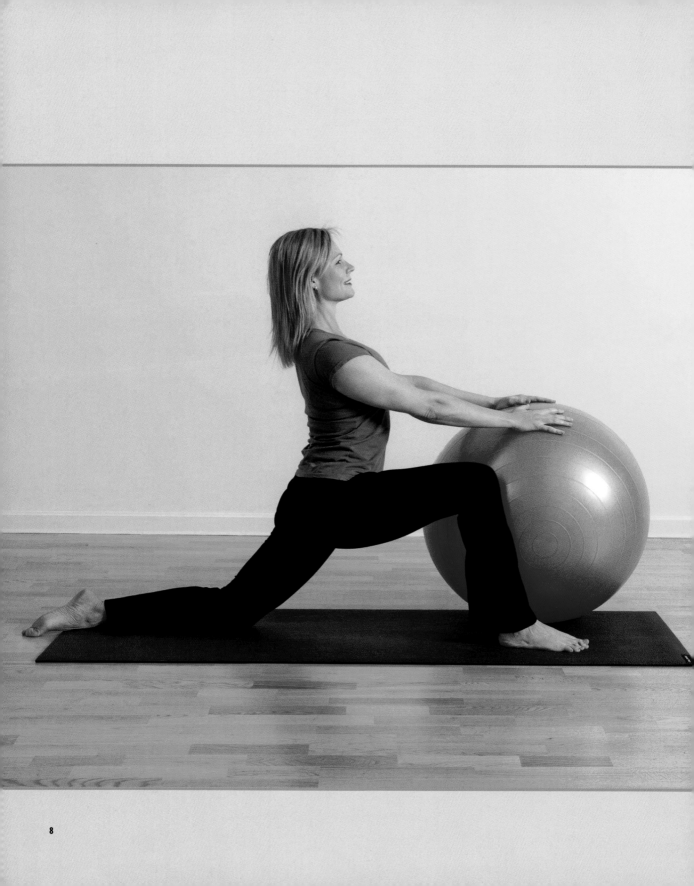

What's The Big Buzz About the Ball?

These days, if you look around gyms, physical therapy clinics, and Pilates studios, you'll most likely see racks of stability balls in various sizes and shapes. Likewise, if you exercise at home, you've probably found the ball to be one of your favorite pieces of equipment.

That's because the stability ball delivers profound results and is easy to use, while also offering a good challenge to both beginners and advanced exercisers. People are completely changing their workout regimens with this user-friendly prop—they do their ab workouts on the ball, lift weights on the ball, and practice yoga and Pilates on the ball!

The ball's effectiveness stems from its ability to naturally establish an awareness of your body's imbalances, thus helping to improve and develop functionality and agility. To translate that to lay terms: because you have to work to keep your balance while you're on the ball, you end up strengthening weak muscles as well as all of your core muscles.

In other words, let's say you do a push-up while on the ball; you not only strengthen your triceps, pectorals, and back muscles as you would with a traditional push-up, but you also add in the extra stabilizing work, so your abs and lower back muscles, as well as all of your smaller supporting muscles get a workout.

But there's more! Anytime you change the way you perform an exercise, you force your muscles to work harder than they're used to. So, once you put that push-up on the ball, your stronger muscles have to work harder than they usually do and your weaker muscles have to pull more of their own weight (if you'll forgive the pun).

As you can see, ball work really can't be beat for both fun and effectiveness.

This is why my clients who work with the ball are hooked! They have reshaped their bodies, look and feel energized, and have dramatically improved their posture. Clients love the ball so much, many of them have begun to use one as the chair at their desks!

The History of the Ball

The Swiss, or stability, ball was originally introduced as the "gymnastic" ball by Dr. Susanne Klien-Vogelbach, a doctor in Switzerland. Dr. Klien-Vogelbach created the ball in the 1960s for use in physical therapy to treat orthopedic and neurological disorders. Doctors had children with cerebral palsy and inefficient motor skill development use the ball to help neuro-muscular stimulation. When someone with poor motor skills uses the ball, their brain pathways are "re-patterned" and they are able to improve the way their body moves.

Swiss ball work began show up on the US physical therapy scene through a protégé of Klien-Vogelbach's. In the '70s and '80s, the ball began to be used as part of the reha-bilitation process for people with spinal injuries.

The first balls were manufactured by an Italian toy manufacturer named Aquilino Cosani, whose company Gymnic remains the leader in ball making. The Gymnic balls became highly acclaimed for helping to develop motor-sensory skills in premature babies and children with traumatic motor-skill retardation. Observers noted that the colorful balls, with their circular shape and dynamic surface, were inviting to the senses while, at the same time, the exercises being done with them produced very positive outcomes.

While the stability ball has always been one of best ways to prevent and rehabilitate injuries, its more likely that you have other goals, such as the long, lean body that comes with Pilates, weight-training, yoga, and other resistance exercise. Fortunately, the ball adds challenge and fun to those exercises—and that's why we're all here! The unstable surface of the ball is the easiest and most foolproof way to become aware of postural deficiencies and then to work to correct them.

Even though ball work was first developed as a form of physical therapy and not as a form of exercise for healthy people, the ball is a natural in the gym! It blends the therapeutic values of stability and balancing skills with conventional exercises while also teaching the importance of using core muscles actively.

Your "core," or center of gravity in your trunk, is made up of your abs, back, and buttocks. The muscles within these body sections need to function together at all times—whether you're just going about your daily activities or you're engaged in an athletic sport or exercise.

For example, on the ball, even if you are doing an exercise focusing on the muscles of your arm, such as doing a biceps curl, your core muscles will still have to support your upper body to maintain good posture and create good muscle coordination as you perform the exercise.

This mindful method develops better-looking, symmetrical, stronger, longer, leaner muscles. This therapeutic approach to exercise is especially important to combat chronic back pain and to avoid unnecessary surgery. The Communication Age requires us to sit and bend forward at computers and driving in cars, in addition to more natural physical requirements, such as lifting children and groceries. And we rarely spend enough time stretching and relaxing our muscles (or strengthening those same muscles in beneficial ways).

The ball's therapeutic benefits come from the shape and unstable surface of the ball in relationship to the natural curves in the spine, which challenges your balance and requires your brain to improve its ability to coordinate your muscles, encouraging more muscles to work together in synergy front to back. The shape of the ball makes it easy to open up tightened rib cages, which improves your breathing and restores elasticity and life to your spine.

Many fitness professionals today use the stability ball in lieu of a weight bench to ensure proper form and to recruit the small stabilizing muscles that provide joint support. Working with the stability ball also conditions the mind as well as the body, allowing you to become aware of how you perform any movement, whether dancing or picking up a baby or playing football. This promotes healthy movement, agility, and injury prevention.

We're fortunate to see those brightly colored balls in all sizes gaining popularity in the fitness world. Many well-educated trainers, some of whom also work in the physical therapy field, continue to develop new ways to incorporate the ball into their repertoire.

Pilates and Ball Work

This is going to sound almost too obvious, but bear with me. If you can't balance on the ball, then you can't really do any sort of exercise properly. Being able to balance means the most important muscles of your body—your core muscles—are strong and capable.

Pilates, a form of exercise developed by Joseph Pilates, will create a strong core. The progressive lessons of Pilates teach postural awareness and correct muscular imbalances. You cannot do ball work without understanding the basics of Pilates.

Today the name Pilates has become a household name in fitness, yet few know the origin of this ingenious exercise form. Joseph Pilates was born in Germany and had been a sickly child determined to overcome an asthmatic condition. He studied yoga, martial arts, circus arts, horseback riding, swimming, and the way animals move—all with an analytical mind.

He worked at a rehabilitation facility for the British army during the war and created a system of exercises using a weight and pulley contraption that the injured could do in bed. He turned hospital beds into therapeutic devices by attaching springs to the bed. His understanding of physics led to his design and production of an eccentric furniture line, which can be viewed in his book, *Your Health* by Joseph Pilates. These pieces are better known today as universal reformers, Wunda chairs, Cadillacs, and wall units, and can be found in all Pilates studios, along with lots of balls! I bet if Joe were alive today he would have created a full program with balls, just like I have.

The Pilates technique stimulates the mind, wakes the body, and helps you to understand your body's "powerhouse," or core. The powerhouse refers to your body's three-dimensional core or center of gravity—basically the muscles of your chest, abs, and back, including the muscles of your upper back, middle back, lower back, and the small muscles that run along your spine. Your body initiates any and all movements from these deep postural muscles, which I will explain in depth later.

Joseph Pilates called his method "contrology," which is shorthand for learning to control your body with your mind.

If you wish to learn the Pilates Method properly, as it was originally taught, you need a concentrated, mindful approach. The same approach is necessary with this ball work.

You need to nurture this technique with practice and patience. This is not just an exercise class to master; it's an education about your body. And once you feel educated and in control of your body, you will also feel more confident.

I have also come to believe that the knowledge and effectiveness that is part of Pilates training keeps people exercising longer and more consistently. The most common reason people give me for not exercising is frustration due to not seeing and feeling results. But this only happens when someone performs their movements recklessly and without proper body awareness. When you exercise properly and understand even a little about body mechanics and postural form, you see and experience immediate results. Then you can also learn how to apply these principals to improve functionality during everyday activities. This experience of results improves your quality of life and encourages lifelong fitness habits.

Get the Inside Scoop

What does core strength mean exactly? When people think about abdominals and abdominal strength, they usually only think about the largest, strongest, and most superficial of the abdominal layers: the "rectus" layer. So, when they exercise, they usually only bend forward.

This is a problem for two reasons. First, the back becomes weaker and weaker as more and more exercises are done in a forward direction. Second, all that movement in one direction shortens the muscles and builds a hard bulge in the belly.

My exercises feature a three-dimensional core focus because the spine can move forward and back, side to side, in a twist, and even up and down. When we move in a way that focuses on the core's three-dimensional ability, then we build true strength, create length and leanness, and aren't in danger of hurting our backs.

I have had countless patients instructed to do crunches by physicians, and their back pain persisted until I developed a new way for them to discover how to effectively use all of their core muscles. Using the ball made the work so much easier for me to teach as well as for them to learn and really understand the concepts. It takes practice, but it's totally worth it!

Working all sides of the trunk restores core balance, allowing all the muscles to gain strength and flexibility. When elasticity is restored, your rib cage works and moves like gills of a fish with every breath. This unlocks your trapped energy, too, and allows you to have more fun. While you're trying out these new exercises, focus on your abs as a whole series of muscles, rather than as a flat muscle that only runs up and down. This new imaging process will allow you to target the deeper core muscles of your body. Your core muscles wrap around and support your middle trunk, connecting and centering your upper and lower body on all levels and sides. These deep muscles do work in conjunction with the superficial rectus to tone, tighten, and help combat chronic back pain.

All of the exercises and visualization in this book will allow you to develop a steady band of support to help you balance on the ball. This enables you to reach deeper layers of your body with new and interesting moves. You won't have to do just crunches anymore!

The Mind-Body Connection

When we exercise regularly, we enjoy the uplifting mental release as well as the physical appearance it provides. When you perform a dance or play a sport or musical instrument, you have to practice with thoughts of how your mind is coordinating with your body to improve each time to win a game, play the right notes, or dance the right choreography. I would like you to approach ball work the same way—with focus and joy!

Following this ball workout regularly and with mindful attention to your form will give you the energized, agile, long, and lean body you have been seeking. Learning how to control your body with your mind enables you to fully benefit from the stability ball workouts. I have personally learned these concepts after physically surviving the school of hard knocks while dancing professionally. "If I knew then what I know now" is the mantra I use to inspire others to reach for longevity and reignite their positive self-image.

A Little Bit About Me

As far back as I can remember, my favorite pastimes consisted of anything that required physical activity, whether taking ballet and tap dancing at age five, playing a competitive sport, riding a horse on the beach, or simply working in the garden with my grandfather. Sunday afternoons were regularly spent singing and dancing or choreographing silly skits with friends after church in my parents' basement.

I managed to convince my parents to accept and fund my desire to become a professional dancer, and I just knew I would succeed against all the odds they continuously reminded me of. I am fortunate that my family lives in a Long Island suburb very close to New York City so I could study there throughout my youth. My intense passion and focus on dance allowed me to be accepted into a performing arts high school, like the Fame school, where half of my school day was spent studying ballet, several modern dance techniques, musical theatre, and Pilates. I had been exposed to a variety of techniques while in high school and looked at several universities that had excellent dance departments. The Alvin Ailey American Dance Center was the school most captivating to me. I loved the raw passion of the Horton technique, and when the live drumming was playing for our mandatory African dance class, the energy would put goose bumps on my arms, it was so special. I still try to find that energy to share with others when I teach my classes seminars and videos. The Ailey School—back when Alvin was still alive—was in the heart of Broadway on 45th Street in the Minskoff Theatre building, so auditions were no problem in between classes. It was mandatory to study Pilates and movement analysis. My teachers were from the old school, and also taught at NYU, Columbia, Julliard, and SUNY Purchase. Dancers are dedicated to their mentors so we would choose schools to study at based upon the faculty.

Eventually, I did end up working as a dancer in videos, dancing with small modern companies, and touring a bit. I wanted to learn every aspect of physical performance, so I trained and worked with circus performers of Ringling Bros. Circus, too. My father was not happy with my choice, but it has proven to be one of the most influential experiences of my work. My sense of adventure and knowledge-seeking taught me to live and to adopt a strong work ethic. Working with the circus was a gift, a truly unique and special experience of learning firsthand from families that for generations have practiced mastering perfect balance, ambidexterity, and unparalleled strength. I learned basic single trapeze and, my favorite, riding no hands bareback on a running elephant. Of course, I was there with my Pilates zeal, training the performers. I loved tutoring the performing children who spoke many languages!

I had a serious chronic ankle injury and used Pilates, as all dancers did, to rehab at a performing arts physical therapy center. The therapy became so interesting to me that it inspired me to go back to school and work towards a physical therapy degree while living in NYC, continuing the dance auditions, and studying a course to become a teacher of Pilates. I studied at the first training centre in NYC, which was called the Institute of Movement Science, with Sean Gallagher, PT, Steve Giordanno, and Romana Kryzanowska—known today as the grand dame of Pilates, having been Joseph Pilates' favorite protégé. He had given Romana his blessing to carry on his studio operations in NYC after his death in the late 1960s. At 83, she is still going strong, and I thank her for being so tough on me and for her generosity of always taking extra time to share her gifts with me.

Romana has incredible intuitive gifts; she has a knowledge of bodies that can't be learned from any textbook. It's only knowledge you can learn first-hand, and I was lucky enough to have the touch of her hands to teach me. I was so lucky to have been one of two apprentices at the time—and no one knew why I was getting up at 5 A.M. every morning to run off to class! I was learning so much more from her than I would have sitting in a classroom that I opted to continue with movement studies instead of mainstream physical therapy.

So, I began to study with Irene Dowd, another genius, who was one of my favorite teachers in the movement science program. She taught neuro-muscular propioception. I later studied anatomy with her as well. When attending her anatomy courses, it's mandatory to bring an artists sketch book and colored pencils to draw the anatomy that you're learning to enhance your sensory understanding. She has inspired my ball classes immensely.

Hard work and study were important to my education, but so was luck! For example, I was fortunate to be touring in Santa Fe, New Mexico with a show when I met Joan Briebart of the Physical Mind Institute in 1991. It was at that moment I knew my life was to remain in this field. She had also studied with Joseph Pilates, only she had become an editor in publishing, not a dancer. Joan is a forward thinking genius in business with an appreciation for what Pilates did for her. She is responsible for bringing Pilates into the mainstream world with her first national course that was developed to allow new students to become certified Pilates teachers.

Joan hired the finest therapists to construct a solid course explaining the anatomical foundations of bio-mechanical movement that make Pilates so special. These courses answered the questions you never asked in NYC—there you just listened to the physical corrections and practiced until you perfected each move. Many other training programs have copied these fundamentals from Joan and adopted them into their own courses. I still teach courses for The Physical Mind Institute and these anatomical foundations have helped me develop cutting-edge progressive programs that change others' lives. I use those words quite frankly.

At the time I was in formal training to become a Pilates instructor, there were no manuals with pictures. We were expected to show up with our artist's notebooks and write in lab notation, or at least our own version of it. This training, coupled with the modern science of Joan Briebart's forward thinking Physicalmind Institute, has established the foundation for me to create this and other progressive courses.

Now, after 20 years, thousands of countless teaching hours, and much time spent seeking out scientific information to prove my theories, Pilates training is still my source of inspiration. I allow my work to evolve in user-friendly ways that will help others fully function in an era of sedentary lifestyles. I teach my unique ball and movement classes at my Insidescoop Studios in New York. And with the belief of my friends at Koch Vision, I have the opportunity to share these ideas on my new Liz Gilles Core Fitness line of videos.

Now it is my job to teach wellness and help others to heal. This is what I was meant to do and it inspires this work! I didn't realize until several years ago that this was a special gift given to me, but my keen intuitive sense kept telling me to follow my heart, stay focused, and face my fears. I listen to mentors carefully and openly, ask lots of questions, and take risks. These are my golden rules or, one might say, mantras I live and work by. Not easy, but so rewarding.

I hope you enjoy this book as much as I have enjoyed sharing it with you. Always follow your heart and be true to your soul!

– Liz

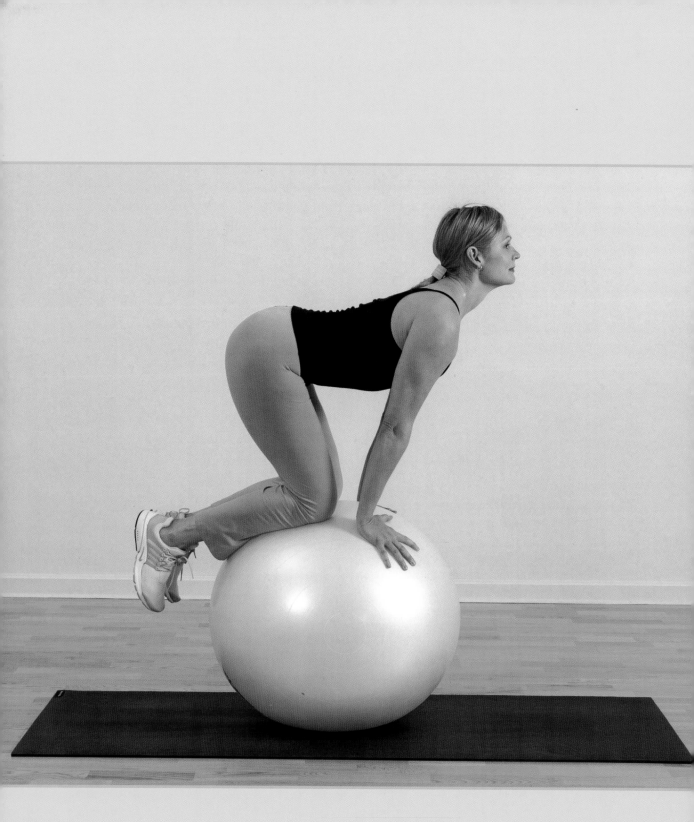

How to Get on the Ball

Before we get started with the exercises, I would like you to get to know your ball so you can ensure maximum benefits and enjoy a safe, effective workout you'll love and want to keep practicing.

How to Pick the Right Size Ball

First, you'll want to make sure that your ball is the proper size for your height. The general guideline is that when you are seated on top of the ball, your thighs should be parallel to the floor when your knees are bent at a right angle. This usually means if your height is less than 5'4", use a 55-cm ball. Fully inflated, the ball should measure 21 inches from top to bottom. If you are 5'5"–6' tall, use a 65-cm ball, which should measure 25 inches from top to bottom.

How to Inflate Your Ball

The quickest and most efficient way to inflate your ball is to take it to the gas station and fill it until it's tight. Don't be afraid of popping the ball, as it can withstand 400 lbs of pressure. The ball may be smaller than you need the first time, but it will stretch over time, so as you use it and it stretches, you can add more air and increase the size based on your needs. Most balls come equipped with a small hand pump and you can also use a bicycle pump. An important point to remember when storing your ball is that significant changes in temperatures will cause the ball to shrink or pop. So, the best way to store your ball (if you're keeping it inflated) is to store it in a climate-controlled space.

How will you know when your ball is inflated to the correct size?

When sitting on your ball, you should ideally have your knees aligned directly above your second toe and your hip bones in line with your kneecaps. Your balance will be challenged because of the dynamic surface of the ball, but you can adjust the tension if you feel nervous that you might fall off. Make sure you are comfortable, as discomfort could be unsafe or make your workout unpleasant.

Use a yardstick to measure the correct height of the ball, since it will have metric measurements on it. You may not feel comfortable balancing on a fully inflated ball because it doesn't have any "give." Here are a couple of modification tips:

1. If want more give in your ball, which will make balancing easier, decrease the tension in the surface of the ball by letting out a little air.

2. Sit lower on the ball.

3. You may want to make your workout more challenging as you improve coordination and mobility. As your body becomes acclimated to the ball, you can add air to harden the surface and sit higher on the ball.

There are variations in ball surfaces depending on the manufacturer. Some balls, such as the Fitball and Gymnics, have a thicker skin than Resist-a Ball or Power Systems, and some are more transparent than others. The thicker skinned balls tend to stretch out a bit after their initial inflation, so you will need to add a bit more air to fully inflate them to their specified size. These balls generally hold their shape longer. The thin-skinned balls stretch out more easily but require frequent pump ups. They are both fine, it's totally up to personal preference. Don't worry; you will bond with your ball before you know it!

Identifying Your
Personal Posture Type

Since the ball helps target deep underpinning muscles that surround the joints, not just the large muscles we typically focus on in exercise, it's important to understand your body and how it works in order to individualize the exercises you're going to do. When these small muscles work together in a synergistic three-dimensional manner, they stabilize joints to enable an extremity or the spine to move more efficiently. Stabilizing muscles are often overlooked and underutilized, unless specifically targeted during exercise, which often happens only in Pilates and yoga. The ball's unstable surface requires you to actively think about these muscles in order to remain stable and balanced. You can't stay on the ball unless you focus!

In fact, before you move in any way on the ball, you have to first engage the core support of your trunk This knowledge creates a body consciousness and awareness so that you become more aware of how your body relies on its core strength to move properly.

Three Key Concepts

There are three key concepts that make these ball moves unique:

1. **Three-dimensional movement:** The unstable surface of the ball forces your body to integrate the postural muscles that encircle your torso to balance, which also increases spinal length and mobility and gives you an aesthetically longer, leaner torso. In other words, these exercises will give you a flat stomach and lifted butt!

2. **Dynamic flexibility:** The ball delivers the subtle balance between strength and flexibility by incorporating both in each exercise. While you're performing each exercise, keep in mind that while the obvious side of the body or muscle is

working, the opposite side is stabilizing for balance, which creates agility and functionality within the muscles. Working this way is more mindful, defines muscles better, and relieves chronic strain and fatigue. This increases your endurance for all other activities.

3. **Functional Movement:** The most important concept to remember while working on the ball is that the ball moves due to its shape and the dynamic surface—and you should too! We will be using the ball as a tool to proprioceptively (meaning how the brain receives information and tells the body how to move) train your body. Remember, muscles do not work in isolation, even when the exercise focuses on just one muscle.

Posture Fundamentals

Proper posture plays a major role in all movement: exercising, dancing, participating in any sport, and functioning with ease and energy everyday!

So, why aren't we all standing tall and pain-free already? Because most of us have postural defects that prevent us from holding our bodies properly and, even more importantly for us, from exercising properly. I'll begin by explaining two common posture types. You will identify the posture you have while standing in front of a mirror, comparing your stance with the characteristics of the two common problem postures: lordosis and kyphosis. There are also flat back, tucked, and swayback postures with no natural curves; 'C' or 'S' curved spines with scoliosis; excessive kyphosis among the elderly; osteoporosis, and combination postures.

We of course are aiming for the "ideal" posture. This means maintaining the natural curves in cervical (neck) and lumbar (lower back) areas with mindfully balanced core muscles working together to form a natural weight belt. This will develop even, strong, and agile core muscles that support both the movements of the spine and the extremities.

My philosophy is if you are teaching or doing an exercise, you should know it's specific purpose, while keeping the entire body in mind. This thought process enables the body to re-pattern muscles to improve balance, strength, flexibility, and posture. My studio has been inundated with patients and clients coming to us who used to train three times a week at the gym. They had assumed that because a machine says it works a particular

LORDOSIS CHECKLIST

Lordosis is when there is a pronounced lumbar or lower back curve. This means that the pelvis is tipped forward or "anteriorly" tilted.

- Weight of the body is over the front of the feet, abdominals hanging forward
- Lower back muscles, buttocks, and lateral hips are very tight due to the tilt
- Hip flexors are tight

KYPHOSIS CHECKLIST

Kyphosis looks like someone is hunched over.

- Mid-back curve is excessive
- Over stretches the hip flexors
- Neck is compressed, causing the chin to fall
- Chest compressing inward
- Common in osteoporosis patients

muscle, that muscle is doing all the work when they begin to move their joints. The truth is, the weight is being imposed upon whichever muscles are posturally available. This may or may not be the muscle(s) they believe will be working. The most common reason for imbalances, chronic pain, and excess bulk in a muscle group, is over-stretched or over-tightened muscles. Everybody's muscles learn how to adopt a comfortable pattern to function together in life based upon spinal posture and joint action, in addition to emotional and dietary input. The stability ball will heighten your postural awareness simply by having to balance! You'll find your ball exercises to be a fun way to get the inside scoop you've always wanted. You will take charge, and be in control of your body, by using your mind.

These fundamental concepts, when applied mentally while performing the physical exercises, teach you anatomical principals you can use everyday. They are the building blocks for any exercise or sport training program. You may want to reread them as you become more accustomed to working with the ball.

You will not only be improving your shape, but also re-patterning muscles, into becoming more functional and efficient. You will improve your awareness by concentrating on opposing or antagonistic muscle groups. The center of gravity in the body is found at the pelvis and rib cage connection—this is the most important thought to have when the core muscles work to hold the spine stable.

These foundations with the ball are designed to bring a conscious level of kinesthetic awareness to the mind, maintaining spinal alignment with stability to promote mobility. Using the ball as a bench to weight train helps to recruit deeper layers of muscles for stabilizing joints and helps you to understand important postural concepts.

OK, take a look at the photos. They demostrate the optimum versus poorly aligned postures in several positions on the ball. The photos of good postures will help you in setting up proper starting positions when beginning each exercise series. Your postural positions and muscular balance will improve with practice, patience, and concentration. Keep in mind—consistancy is key. Slow and steady progress will make your workout a natural part of your life, just like brushing your teeth!

You want to mindfully set up each starting posture with a neutral spine. This term refers to the alignment of your joints and spine. Finding your center of gravity in each exercise helps you develop balance and coordinate your muscles on both the front and back of your body. This allows even engagement of the muscles recruited for each movement. Although a neutral position can be identified in many joints simultaneously, we will concentrate on the most significant—the pelvis—to begin.

The pelvis is the body's center of power. The pelvis lines up like a triangle between the two predominant bones near the top of the pelvis—the ASIS (anterior superior iliac spine) and the pubis, or pubic bone. We want to prevent the top of the pelvis from rocking either too far forward or too far back, but instead remaining centered to coordinate the core muscles between the rib cage and pelvis.

Proper Sitting Pose

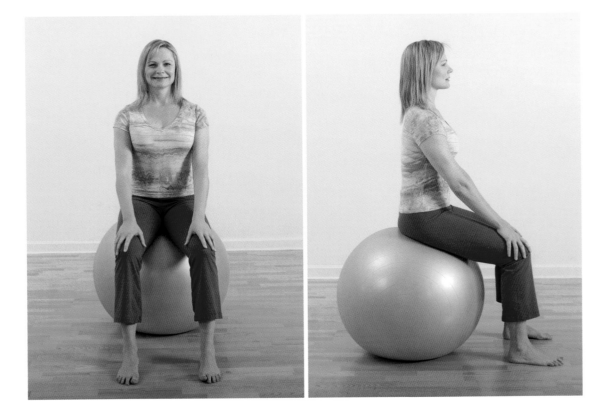

- If you look at your body from the side, your shoulders and hips should be "stacked," or in line with each other.

- Your butt should be just below the apex, or top point, of the ball, with a tripod of your tailbone and two "sitting bones" creating even and relaxed weight distribution.

- The crease line of your hip and your knees should be in a straight line.

- Your ankle should be in line with your knees.

Over-Tucking with Posterior Tilt

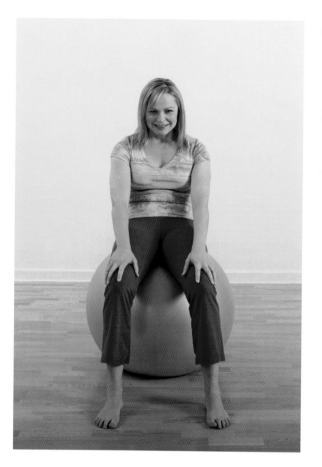

● This posture overworks the front thighs and compresses your lumbar spine. It makes your chest round too much and your head jut forward.

● You'll need to concentrate on bringing your tailbone back and bending your knees at the hip to elongate your hamstrings. Think of creating space in your trunk by lifting your rib cage upward, stretching your abs and back instead of crunching in the middle. Adjust your skull backwards by pulling the rounded area in the back of your skull straight back. Be careful not to confuse this action with lifting your chin up or squashing the front of your neck down. This may require a bit of practice. Make your neck long by lifting through the back of your head.

Over-Arched Lumbar Spine

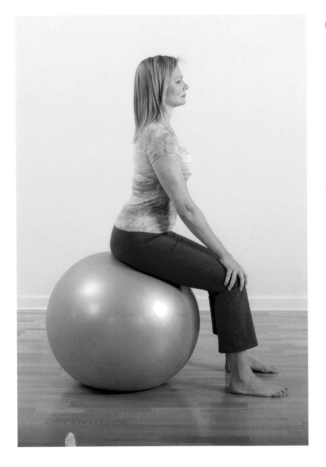

○ The tendency is to tilt your pelvis forward and bring your body with it, so that you're almost leaning forward from the hips. This makes your abdominals hang forward and overuses the muscles of your lower back and shoulders. Instead, try to sit squarely on your hips and sit bones.

○ Keep the weight of your trunk back on your pelvis tripod. This may feel unnatural, as if you're leaning back, but as you work your core abs, back, and hips together, your trunk muscles will begin to synchronize and eventually it won't feel comfortable to lean forward anymore!

Proper Prone Position

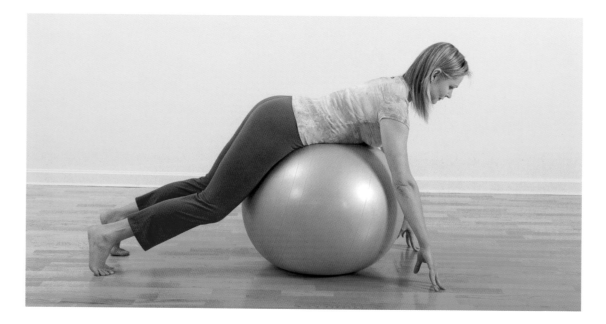

● Your should have a neutral pelvis with your rib cage resting just beyond the apex of the ball. You want your knees bent, thighs resting against the ball to prevent the tendency to tuck and over-use the muscles on the front of your body. You may think that because you're lying on your belly, you'll automatically work you back body muscles. Surprise, but no! Your strong front muscles are sneaky, and will take over regardless of position, unless you take charge.

● Your toes should be bent under towards the ball with your weight distributed evenly across all ten toes. Stretch from the ball of your feet through your arches to relay a lifted feeling up through the back of your thighs. Lift up with your butt muscles. Your neck should be long with your shoulder blades sliding gently toward your spine to control your arm placement and provide shoulder stability. This position is the toughest to "feel" so try and relax and think about the placement of your body.

Over-Tucked
Prone Position

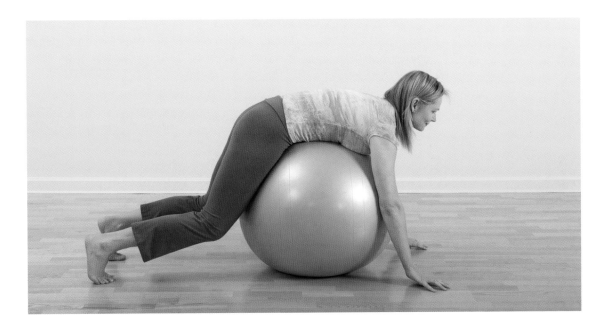

● In an over-tucked position your back will be rounded and your neck will feel strained.

● Your thighs jam into the ball and when you try to move onto your toes with bent knees your body tends to tuck more.

● In all the starting positions, this one in particular, you need to remember the most important point is to stretch the front of your body to target those weak, over-stretched back extensor muscles.

● Keep thinking of your belly button actively up and in to create space between your rib cage and pelvis, encouraging your back muscles to engage, while your hip flexors relax in the front body.

Lying Supine on the Ball

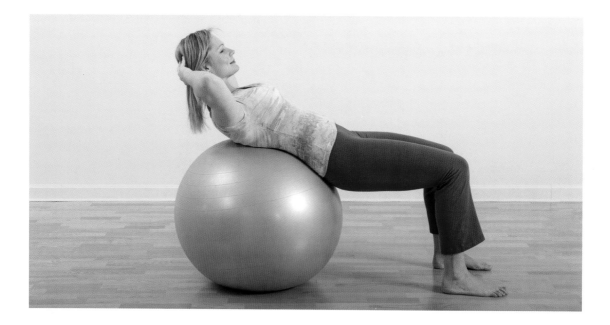

○ Begin by sitting on the ball. Slowly walk your feet forward with your hands supporting you on the ball, until your lower back rests on the ball. Your hands can be placed behind your head to release strain on your neck. If you are in the correct position, your neck should feel free. Your ankles should align directly under your knees, your thighs parallel to one another and the floor.

○ If you are over-arched, your back muscles are already tight. You'll need to elongate your front thighs by really bringing your buttocks to the ball.

○ You need to feel the connection between your ribs and pelvis in this position. Your rib cage needs to press into the ball and the back of your head drops into your fingertips. Your gaze focuses forward.

○ Widen the space between your tight shoulder blades and encourage your rib cage to close and lower to meet your pelvis.

Side Lying over Ball

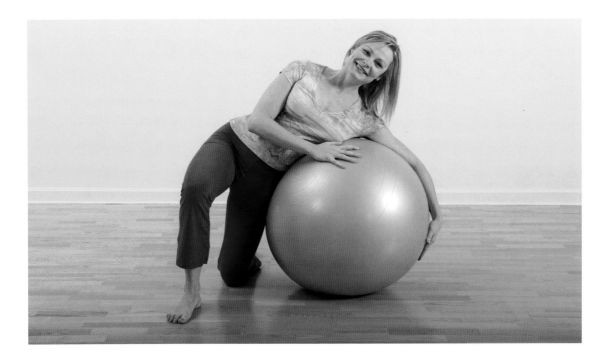

- This is one of the trickiest positions to get used to. The trunk is used to flexing and extending in daily activities, but not used to bending laterally. The muscles surrounding the rib cage become tight and lose the elasticity for side bending, as well as rotating. By the way, spinal rotation is the only movement of the spine that actually nourishes it. This is why rotations are the basic elements in yoga and in my ball work too!

- So, to get set up in a side lying position over the ball, hug the ball into one hip with the elbow of the arm that's on the ball pointing up to the ceiling.

- Try to lift and separate your rib cage over the ball. Use your outside hand on the ball for support, and when your body becomes acclimated, you can try to put both hands behind your head.

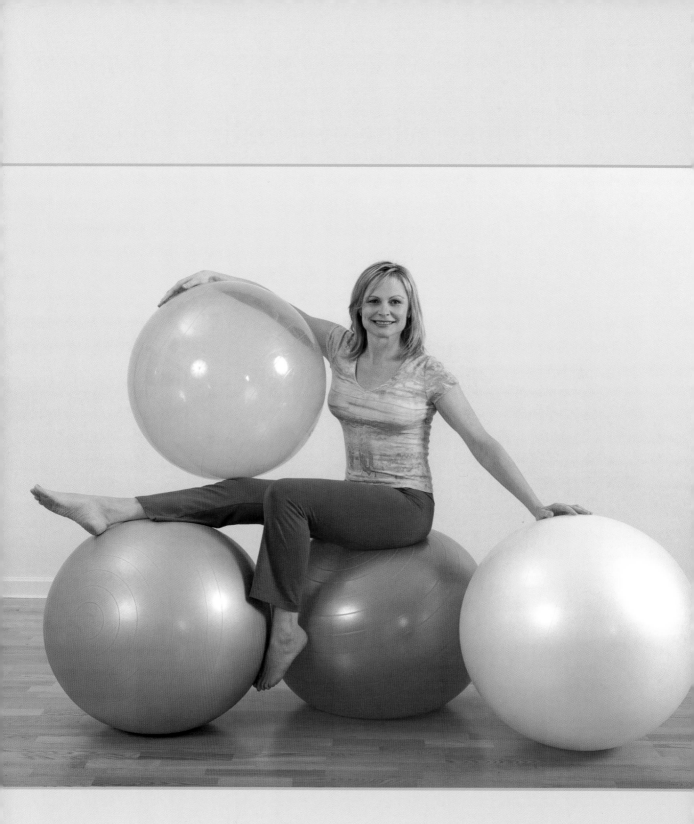

Bonding with Your Ball—The Warm-Up

S o, now we begin the series of exercises. Have patience when starting, even if you're used to working out regularly. This ball workout is a great way to learn how the body works three-dimensionally. Continue working with the thought process of tightening superficial muscles to the max on every rep and exercise. If you do not know how to regulate this, try to think about the synergy of your core and extremities working in a beautiful relationship. Honestly, the ball's unstable surface will remind you! The ball will keep you interested, coming back to challenge a balance or stretch.

You may find it difficult to perform some of these exercises, so try to stay with one level until your body adapts. Initially, you might feel the ball is too big, but stick with it. Try thinking about the opposing primary muscles being worked by pressing into the ball, targeting opposite stabilizers, and creating a fabulous dynamic workout that will make you feel accomplished, inspired, and looking better than ever!

We begin each class with a nice spinal warm-up so your mind connects with where your body is on that day. Use this time to focus your mind; each time you perform a series you will become more at ease using the ball. Think of these as rhythmic warm-up exercises which are fun and release tension. Put on your favorite CD and have fun!

1 Round and Arch

BENEFITS: Warms up the lower back and abs.

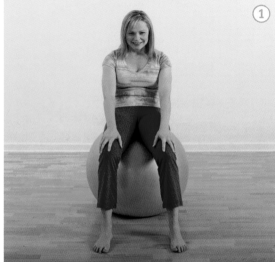
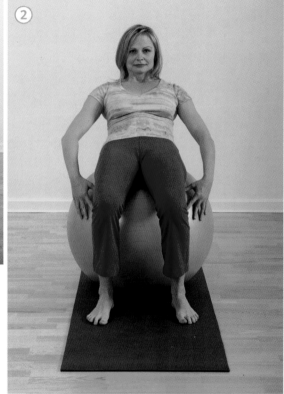

(1) Sit on the ball and scoop up your pelvic floor muscles. Tighten your "bathroom muscles" and feel a lift upward in your abs. Continue up through your ribs, and inhale after your muscles are engaged.

(2) Roll the ball forward, keeping your knees bent over your ankles, rounding your pelvis under with the goal of using your abs to scoop and lengthen your tailbone under until your sacrum touches the ball.

(3) Exhale as you roll your pelvis back through the neutral position into an arched position. Your abs are still actively engaged upward to support the spine. Do this 6 times each way with your hands on the ball for support.

2 Lateral Hip Stretch

BENEFITS: Opens and stretches the hips.

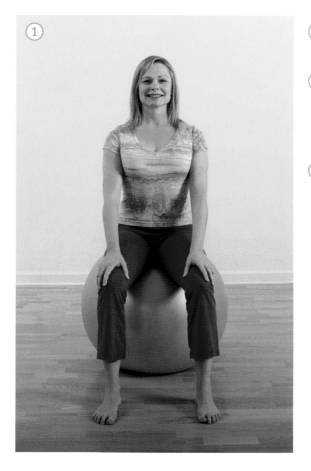

(1) Sit on the ball, your ankles under your knees, feet firmly planted on floor.

(2) Lift your abs up before moving your hip out to the side from the buttocks. Contract your thigh muscles to keep your knees aligned and parallel.

(3) Stretch to the opposite side and notice if you feel more tension in one hip than the other. Use natural breathing so you will stay focused on initiating the pelvic floor and deep core muscles. Repeat 4 times.

Make sure both hips and buttocks stay
even on the ball.

3

Upper Body Arm Swings

BENEFITS: Stretches the shoulders, chest, and back.

(1) Sit tall on top of the ball with your arms at your sides.

(2) Inhale, expanding your ribs as you roll the ball forward. Swing your arms loosely up, stretching your lats and abs.

(3) Roll the ball back and exhale, releasing your arms loosely down to your sides, maintaining a tall torso, with your knees stacked over your ankles. Each rep should stretch your muscles further. Repeat 6 times.

Make sure you're actively lifting your abs as if you're stretching the skin of your abs up. Try not to move from the shoulders. Instead, move with your chest and back muscles for stability and strength.

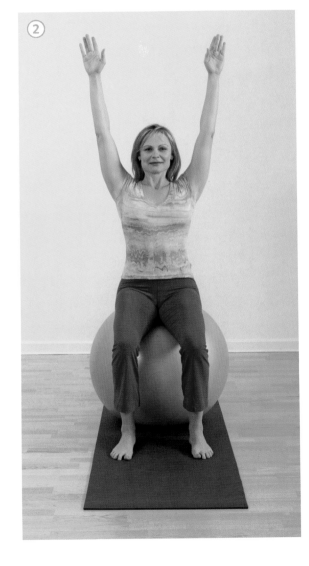

Upper Body Stretch

BENEFITS: Opens the shoulder and neck joints.

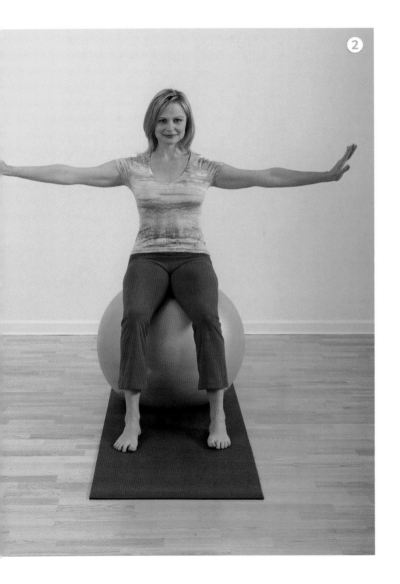

① Sit on the ball with your arms out straight from your shoulders.

② Inhale as you open your chest and slide your shoulder blades in towards your spine as you stretch your arms out. Pulse your arms back 2 times.

③ Exhale, round your back, and pulse 2 times inward, scooping up your abs to open your shoulder blades. Your pelvis stays neutral. Repeat 6 times.

Feel your rib cage lift off your pelvis in back instead of dropping.

5 Single Sliding Arm Side Stretch

BENEFITS: Lengthens your side muscles and opens your ribs.

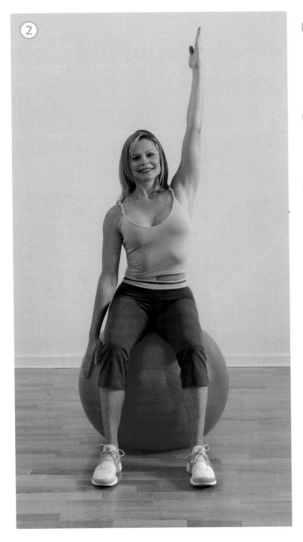

(1) Sit on the ball and extend your left arm up straight, palm facing in. Your right arm is down against the ball, palm facing in with a straight elbow.

(2) Pull down with your right arm as you extend your left arm up and over your torso (this decompresses the rib cage.)

(3) Come back to center, re-engage your abdominals, and repeat on the other side. Do 4 times.

The palm on the ball should slide down with slight pressure to help keep your opposite hip down. This will allow you to feel your obliques work to keep your core stable and your spine upright.

6

Full Spinal Flexion

BENEFITS: Relaxes and stretches the back and neck.

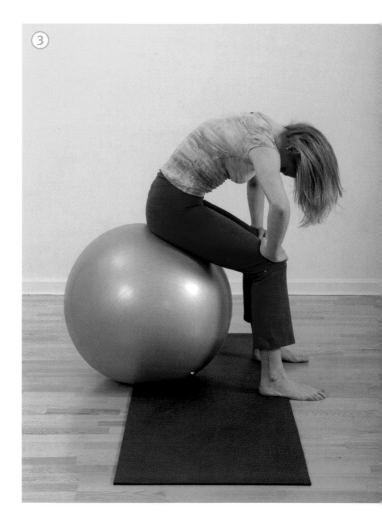

① Sitting tall on the ball, brace your hands on top of your thigh bones.

② Lengthen your spine from the top of your head. Lift your deep abdominal muscles with a soft scooping feeling and bend forward, rounding your spine over your thighs. The ball will roll forward to perpetuate the spinal fluidity. Drop your head down to look at the floor.

③ Press on your hands to help your abs scoop again and roll the ball back, rolling your spine one vertebra at a time from base to skull to a sitting position. Repeat 4 times.

If your balance is challenged, keep the ball roll movements small initially. Progress slowly and steadily to gain the best results.

Torso Twist on Ball

BENEFITS: Releases the side abdominal muscles (obliques).

(1) Sit on the ball with your arms crossed and your knees and hips in a straight line. Your ankles should be under your knees.

(2) Use your abdominals to lift your rib cage off your hips as you breathe in.

(3) Rotate your trunk to the left, making sure your elbows stay in a rectangle shape. As your rib cage moves left, think of your pelvis staying forward—almost imagine an opposing pull to keep your hips square.

(4) The head softly turns with your spine, glancing back, keeping your neck long.

(5) Return to the center and repeat on the other side. Do 3 times each way.

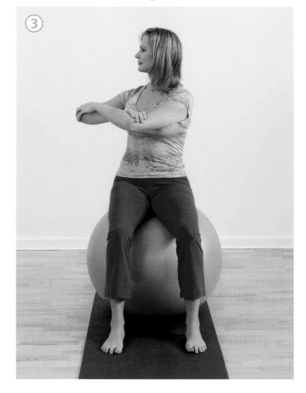

Make sure your knees stay straight forward in line with your hips. If your legs begin to move, this indicates your pelvis is also moving, which compromises spinal length. Begin with a small twist, but use intense concentration for lifting. Use your breathing to keep length in your spine and to recruit your obliques.

Standing and Side Lying Moves

Standing exercises improve balance and coordination, as well as help you break a sweat and get your entire body in shape. I developed a lot of these moves as a way to add circular motions to exercises we do with our joints that can rotate. We tend to move in a linear fashion, treating ball and socket joints as hinges, but the ball is a perfect tool to explore the possibilities and abilities of our muscles and joints. Some of these exercises reflect that thought process; some are just plain fun, but they are all completely effective and easy to learn. Enjoy!

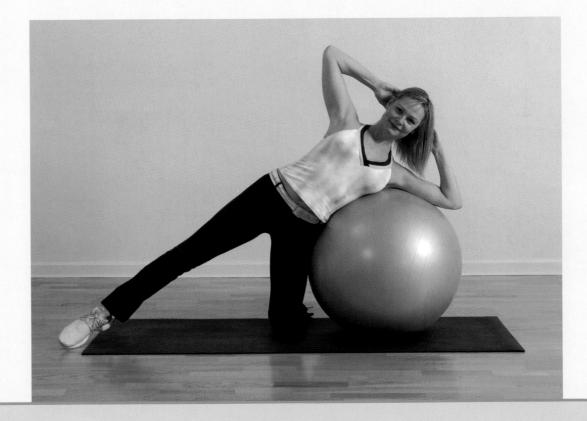

8

Standing Lat Stretch

BENEFITS: Counteracts the rounding of the back that can occur when you sit in front of a computer or at the steering wheel for too long.

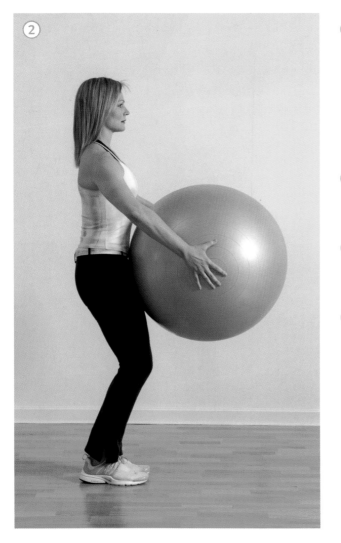

① Stand with your legs together, knees softly bent. Hold the ball with both hands, keeping your shoulders blades wide and down. Your chest and back should feel strong and lifted. Make sure your abs are scooped and lifted.

② Squeeze the ball firmly with the heels of your hands, keeping our fingers soft.

③ Lifting from your mid-back, extend the ball overhead. Keep your shoulders down and steady.

④ Return the ball back to your thighs, maintaining a straight back. Do 5 times.

9

Standing Lateral Side Bend

BENEFITS: Stretches the entire side body while strengthening your front torso and back muscles.

 Stand with your legs just past hip-distance apart, feet slightly turned out, knees slightly bent. Hold the ball in your hands; keep your shoulders down and relaxed.

② Lift the ball overhead with straight arms and bend to one side.

③ Return to center, repeat on other side. Do 2 times on each side.

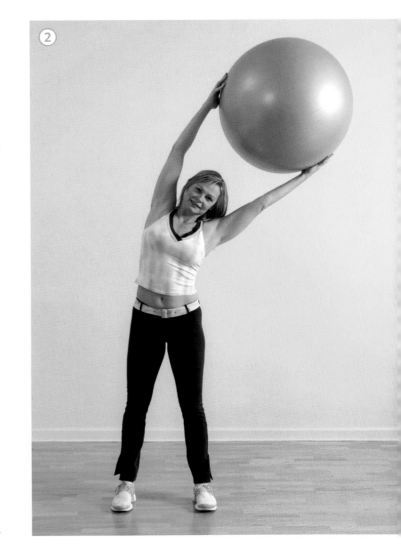

Engaging the proper core muscles prior to bending will give you a tiny waist. But if you clench your muscles, you'll get both a thick waist and a compressed lumbar spine, so stay relaxed even though you are engaging your muscles. It's key to make sure your shoulders are in line with your hips, not swaying behind. Keep your legs bent, but as you get stronger, you can straighten them prior to raising back to center on each side.

10

Semi-Circle Arm Twists

BENEFITS: Tones and stretches your waist, upper back, and arms.

① Stand with your legs hip-distance apart, knees bent.

② Hold the ball at your waist, hands on either side (top and bottom) of the ball. You should be able to see your chest over the ball—this will ensure scapula stability and mobility.

③ Lift your elbows to engage the chest muscles.

④ Twist the ball from side to side, leading with your elbows and reaching from your scapula (shoulder blades).

⑤ Keep your hips very still, engaging your lower abs, but not squeezing your butt, which will compromise the chest and upper body placement. Do this 8 times on a count of 3 or 4.

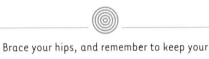

Brace your hips, and remember to keep your back straight, finding your center of gravity. Try not to sway your rib cage forward or back.

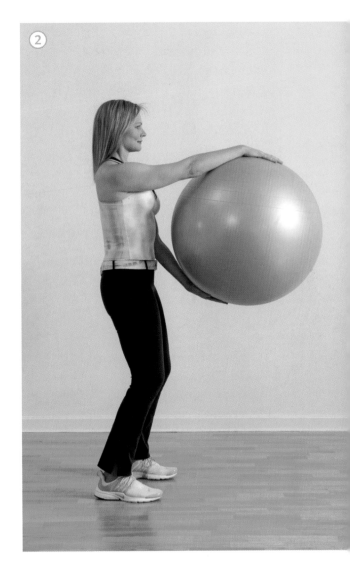

②

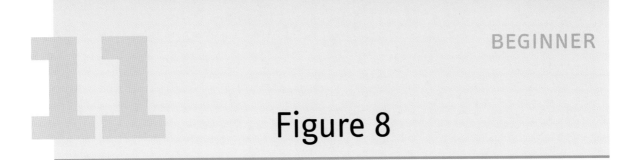

Figure 8

BENEFITS: Restores range of motion to your upper back and shoulders.

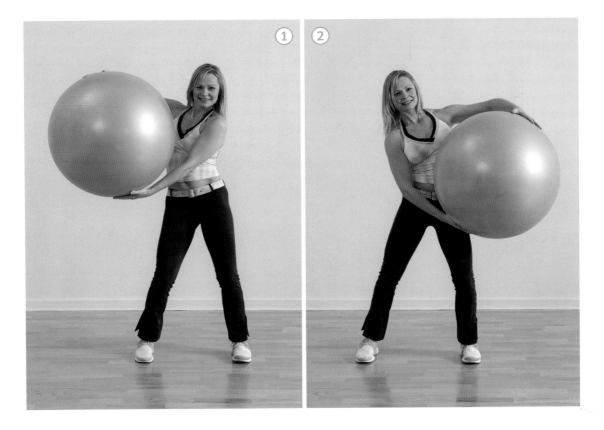

(1) Stand with your legs hip-distance apart, knees bent. Hold the ball with both hands at waist-height. You should be able to see your chest over the ball. Lift your elbows to engage your chest muscles, or pectorals.

(2) Move the ball in a swooping figure-8 shape, beginning at one shoulder and changing direction at your pelvis. The ball should stay within the frame of your shoulders and hips. Repeat 6 times.

12 Rolling Front Lunge

BENEFITS: Stretches your hips flexors (the muscles that run from the bottom of your torso to your upper thigh) and hamstrings, while working your quadriceps.

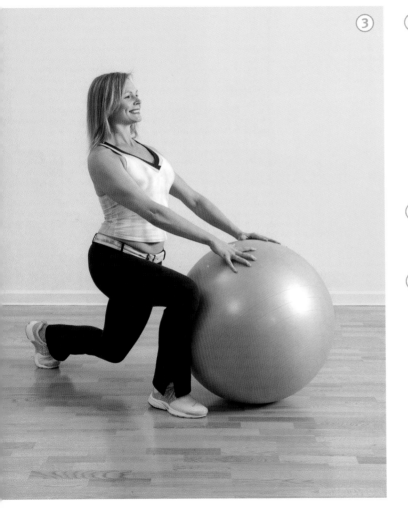

③

① Stand in a parallel lunge position with about two feet between your front and back legs. Your weight should be on the ball of your back foot. The ball is just ahead of your right leg. Squeeze your knee firmly against the ball to feel the inner thigh and trunk lift off the legs.

② Now, engage your core muscles and evenly distribute the weight of your body over both legs.

③ Bend both knees simultaneously, as the ball rolls forward, keeping your spine straight over your legs. Do 6 times on each side.

13 Rolling Spine Stretch

BENEFITS: Stretches your whole back.

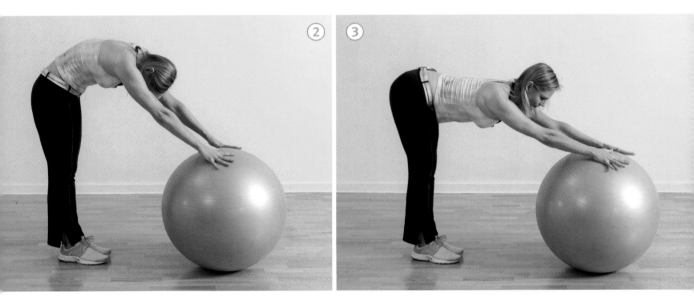

1. Stand behind the ball, feet together, with your back thighs firmly held together. Your knees can either be bent or straight, depending on your hamstring flexibility. Your weight should be distributed evenly on both feet. Round forward and put your hands on the ball with straight arms.

2. Roll the ball forward, keeping your spine rounded, slowly releasing one vertebra at a time until your arms extend, and you feel the stretch in your lats and hamstrings. Feel as if you're pulling taffy.

3. Pull the ball back with straight arms, keeping your shoulder blades engaged, and then use your abs and hamstrings to roll up to a standing position. Do 5 times.

14 Twisting Spiral Lunge, Hand on Hip

BENEFITS: Strengthens your iliotibial band, which runs along the outside of your thigh.

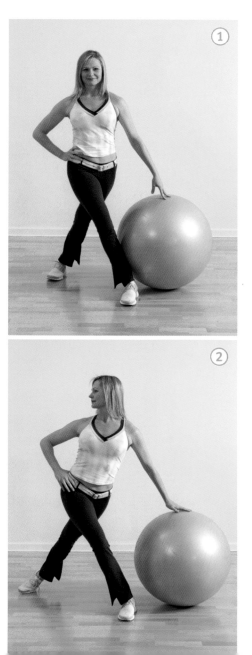

① Stand straight and take a big step forward with one foot—at least a leg's length. Turn your back toes in and your front toes out, so your feet are parallel. Keep your hips facing forward and allow your knees to flex gently as your back heel lifts off the floor. Hold the ball behind your front heel with your finger tips and put your opposite hand on your hip.

② Initiate the move by bending your front knee as that hip rotates backwards. At the same time, your straight arm rolls the ball forward, keeping your spine lifted off your hip and using your abs and outside thigh together to lift as knee bends forward. Your elbow and trunk twist back at the same time.

③ Roll the ball back, do several reps, and, on the last rotation, hold the twist to maximize the stretch. Change sides, taking a moment to feel the difference in the length of your legs. Repeat 3 times each way.

15

Extended
Spiral Lunge

BENEFITS: Strengthens your iliotibial band, which runs along the outside of your thigh.

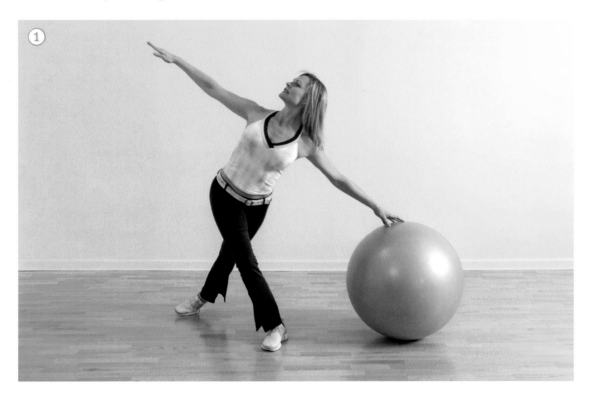

(1) From Twisting Spiral Lunge, continue extension, lunging deeper and extending arm straight behind you.

(2) Repeat 8 times up and down. Hold at the top and and pulse down 8 counts.

Lift your trunk straight up and off the ball as if posting on a horse.

16 Ball Wall Squats

BENEFITS: These wall exercises are great for skiers. They develop balanced strength as well as an awareness about spinal alignment. They also improve postural form, and stabilize your spine, so you can concentrate on engaging muscles to work dynamically around the thighs while lifting your abs. This allows your body to work with foolproof efficiency, instead of dropping weight downward into your knees and ankles. Don't worry if you only feel front thighs work when performing traditional squats.

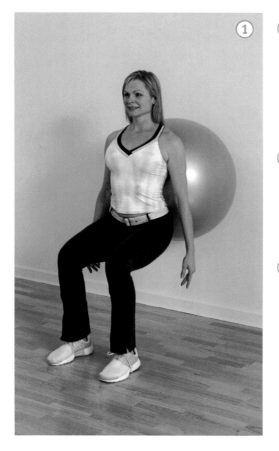

1. Stand against a wall with the ball centered between your upper and lower back. Lean back into the ball, bending your knees into a 90-degree right angle (table top stance) with neutral pelvic placement.

2. The ball will feel as if it's rolling up the wall as the body goes down. Keep your spine pressed into the ball, using your abs to scoop. Remain very straight and stop when your knees are even with your hips.

3. Roll back up to your original starting position. Repeat 6 times, adding a ten-second hold on the last two.

As your strength improves, hold the bend position longer before returning back to the starting position. If your have knee problems, limit the bend until your legs get stronger.

17

2nd Position Grande Plié

BENEFITS: Strengthens and lengthens the hamstrings (back of thighs) and quads (front of thighs), as well as sculpts the butt.

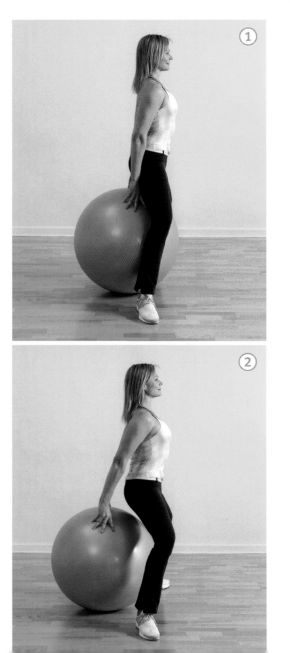

(1) Stand in front of the ball in a wide dancer second position, legs turned out from your hips. Use your hands to hold the ball directly behind your hips.

(2) Use your abs and back to keep a neutral pelvis with upward lift. As you bend your knees into a deep plié—tracking each knee out on line over the second toe—use your arms to roll the ball behind with straight elbows. Do this 8 times.

Engage your abdominals and feel the control come from your hips as you lower your torso. And, as you're doing so, try to press your knees back further to open from the hips and buttocks. Lean back slightly into your hands to feel your triceps engage. Pull your shoulders away from your ears to stabilize and open your chest.

18

Squats

BENEFITS: Shapes and tones the butt and thighs.

① Stand in a wide parallel stance with the sides of your thighs pulling upward and inward to engage your hips and protect your lumbar spine. Your abs should be lifted in and up.

② Hug the ball into your chest so the spine will stay straight.

③ With your weight pulling backwards into your buttocks, lower to a wide plié position, keeping your chest lifted and extending your arms overhead. Keep your spine as straight as possible, knees bent, tracking over second toe as you lower and lift. Do this 8 times.

Keep your spine straight by feeling your chest lift up as it assists your arms in lifting the ball.

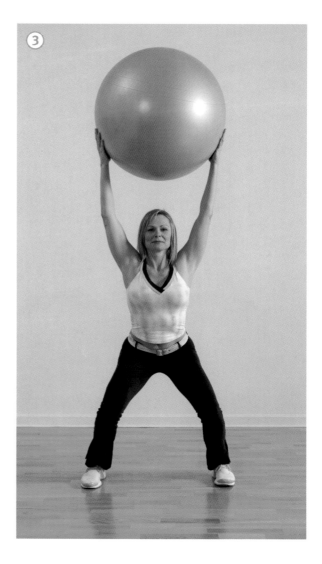

19

Perfect Lunges:
Front Ball Hug

BENEFITS: I developed my famous ball lunges in an effort to deliver the feeling of working muscles with dynamic oppositional pull to re-pattern faulty gait patterns and develop the iliotibial band, which runs along the outside of the thigh.

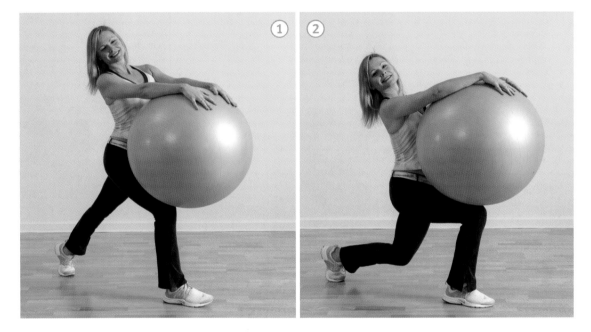

① ②

① Stand with your legs one in front of the other (wide parallel stance) and bend your front knee into a lunge position. The ball should be hugged against your bent front thigh. Raise your back heel to stretch your arch. Your weight should be on the underside of your toes. Pay attention to keeping your ankles even and your hips squared.

② Place your forearms on top of the ball and press downward. Feel your chest rise up as your abdominals lift and stretch, elongating your spine and locking in proper hip alignment. Lower to a deep lunge position then rise back up. Move slowly, 3 counts each way. Repeat 6 times on each leg. Perform two sets.

20 Frog Jumps

BENEFITS: Builds strength in the entire leg.

(1) Stand with your legs wide apart and turn your toes out. Place the ball on the floor in front of you. Bend deeply at the knees until you can place your hands around the ball with your elbows pressed into the inside of your thighs to help stretch them open. Use your buttocks and abs to lift your weight off your knees.

(2) Using the power in your thigh muscles, arches, and buttocks, jump into the air, simultaneously lifting the ball overhead. Point your toes and really straighten your legs in the jump for the most advanced explosive plyometric movement—great for training professional skaters or any other sport requiring explosive moves. Repeat 5-8 times.

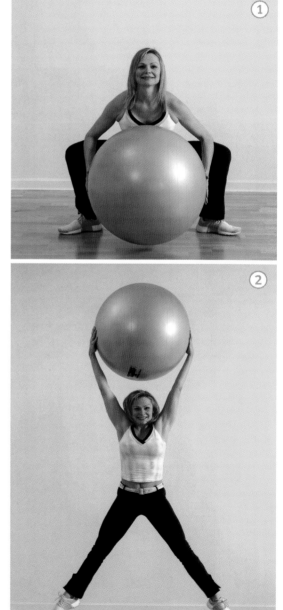

Propel the ball upward as your feet push firmly off the floor using your arches. Be sure to land "toe-ball-heel" using your abs to help your back muscles hold your trunk upright. Don't allow your knees to collapse inward. Use your outer hip and buttocks to control your knees. If your spine is seriously degenerated, don't do this exercise if it's new to you.

21

Standing Back Hip Extensions

BENEFITS: Develops upper back strength while totally lifting your butt.

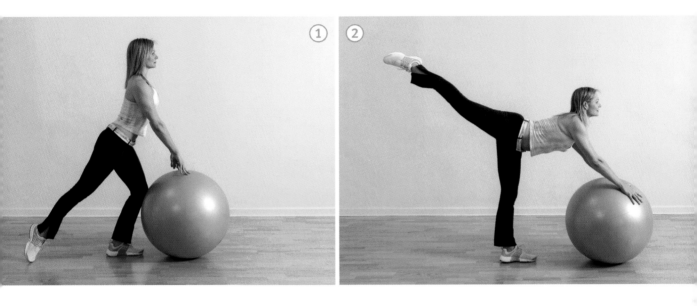

(1) Stand with the ball in front of your knees with both hands on top of the ball. One knee bends against the ball while your straight arms pull the ball against your knee to create the opposition to engage the upper back and scapula for stability.

This is advanced. Start with fewer reps initially and build up. Make sure your arms are pulling the ball towards your body so your back and abs work together to hold your chest up.

(2) Lift your other leg, keeping it as straight as possible, up to hip level. Keep your hips level if possible, to establish the stretch on the side of your hip and thigh that are supporting your body. Straighten your bottom leg and roll the ball out in front of you as you stretch your torso out long. Hold your top leg up, pointing and flexing your ankle joint and activating your calf as well. Do this 4 times. Repeat with your other leg.

22 Standing Front Leg Lifts

BENEFITS: Improves your posture while strengthening and lengthening your leg muscles.

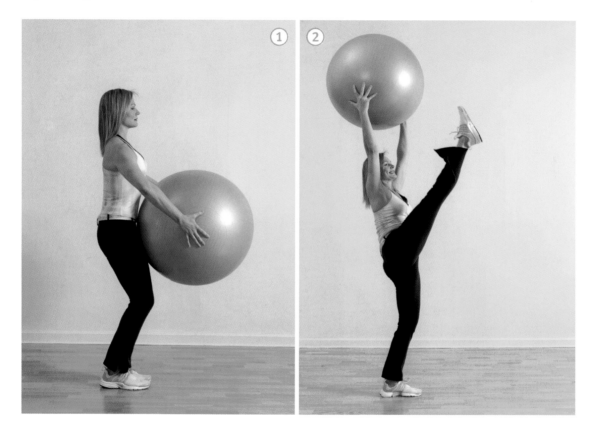

(1) Stand with your legs together in a parallel position. Hold the ball with your arms down.

(2) Lift the ball over your head as you kick one leg up as high as you can in front

of you. Use the ball to encourage your core to keep your pelvis and rib cage connected as your leg is moving off the floor. Extend your knee straight as you kick. Repeat 8 times with each leg.

23

2nd Position with Tricep Dips

BENEFITS: This is a great example of a compound exercise—it works more than one muscle at a time. The main focus is on the back of your arms—the triceps muscle—but because you're standing in a turned out position (like a ballerina) you're also engaging your butt muscles and inner thighs.

(1) Stand in front of the ball, legs spread about two or three feet apart and legs turned out from the hips about forty-five degrees. Your knees should be pointing over your toes (although ideally you can see your big toe when you bend your knees).

(2) Place your hands on the ball, directly under your shoulders, fingertips point toward your butt. Lift your heels off the floor and put your weight on the balls of your feet with arches stretched.

(3) Use your abs and back to keep a neutral pelvis and maintain an upward lift through your spine as arms bend and straighten. Use your triceps to lower and raise your body, holding the ball in place. Do this 8 times.

(4) Next, raise your heels up and keep your elbows straight as you pulse up and down, rolling the ball back and forth. Do this 8 times.

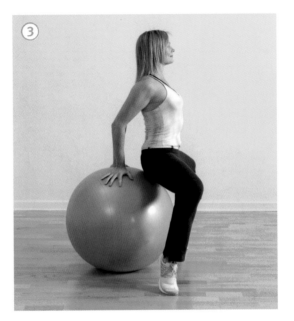

(5) Lower your heels to the floor and keep your elbows straight as you bend your knees into a deep plié without raising your heels off the floor. Keep your knees pressed back. Do 8 times.

Be sure to pull your shoulders away from your ears to stabilize and open your chest.

ADVANCED

24 Full Twisting Two-Handed Spiral Lunge

BENEFITS: This is almost like doing a one-legged squat and I think it's the most effective butt exercise there is.

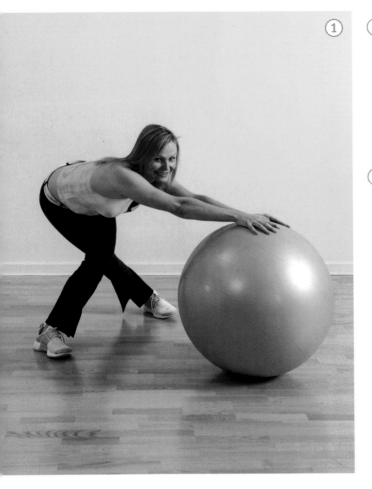

① **Stand in a curtsy position, your right leg straight and your left knee bent and crossed in front of your right leg. Your torso faces forward with both feet parallel. The heel of your right foot is up, with your weight forward on the toes and heel of your left foot.**

② **Hold the ball in front of the thigh of your left leg. Then sweep the ball across your body with straight arms in a circular motion as your hips lift and pull backwards. Continue moving front to back, feeling your hips open. Do this move 4-6 times, then hold and pulse for 8 counts in the curtsy position, then repeat to other side.**

Your arches should be active in any lunges to facilitate proper weight distribution. This will send energy up through the upper most part of your inner thighs, as if you have to go to the bathroom and are holding it.

25 Side Bend with Straight Leg Side Lift

BENEFITS: Slims the outer thighs and, at the same time, you have to really use your obliques to keep your body aligned. You'll notice a real difference in your posture and in the curve of your waist.

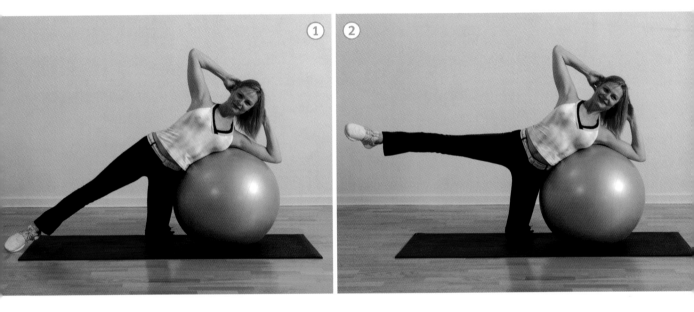

①   Begin on two knees. Hug the ball into one hip while moving your rib cage over the ball. Contour the space between your rib cage and pelvis into the ball and lean sideways over the ball with your hands behind your head.

②   Straighten the leg that's away from the ball, then lift it up to hip-height, while still hugging the ball into your waist with your arm and side. Try not to allow your hips and pelvis to move away from the ball.

③   Lower your leg back to floor. Do 5 times. Switch sides.

26 Straight Leg with Circles

BENEFITS: Strengthens your outer thigh muscles (the abductors).

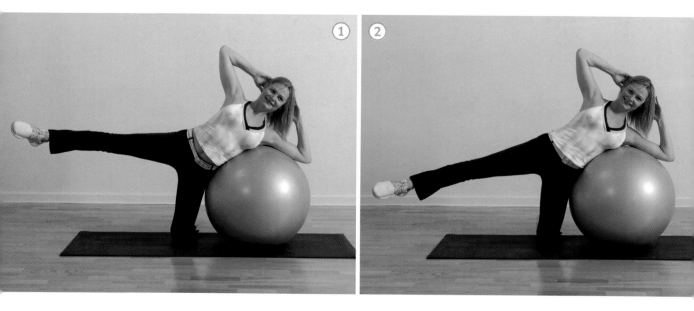

(1) Begin on two knees. Hug the ball into one hip while moving your rib cage over the ball. Contour the space between your rib-cage and pelvis into the ball and lean sideways over the ball with your hands behind your head.

(2) Straighten the leg that's away from the ball, then lift it up to hip-height, while still hugging the ball into your waist

with your arm and side. Try not to allow your hips and pelvis to move away from the ball. Circle your straight leg backwards from your hip.

(3) Circle your leg forwards.

(4) Lower your leg to the floor. Repeat 5 times. Switch sides and repeat.

27

Chest and Arm
Reach and Twist

BENEFITS: Opens your chest, especially if you have a tendency to hunch over your desk or steering wheel. It's also a great release for tight shoulders.

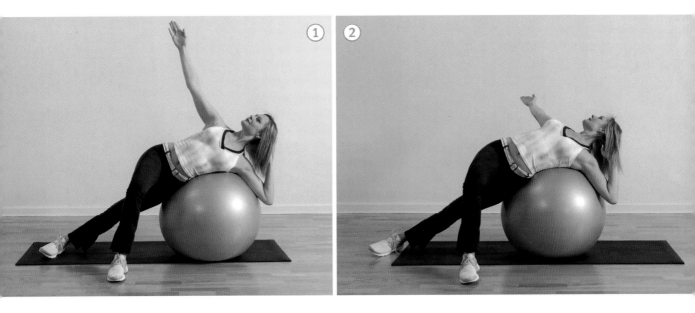

① Begin lying on your side on top of the ball with your bottom leg straight, and your top leg crossed over your bottom leg. Your bottom arm is bent behind your head and your top arm is straight up from your shoulder, palm facing forward.

② Twist your rib cage to the ceiling and open your chest, circling your arm back.

③ Complete the arm circle as your body returns to the starting position. Do 5 times. Switch sides and repeat.

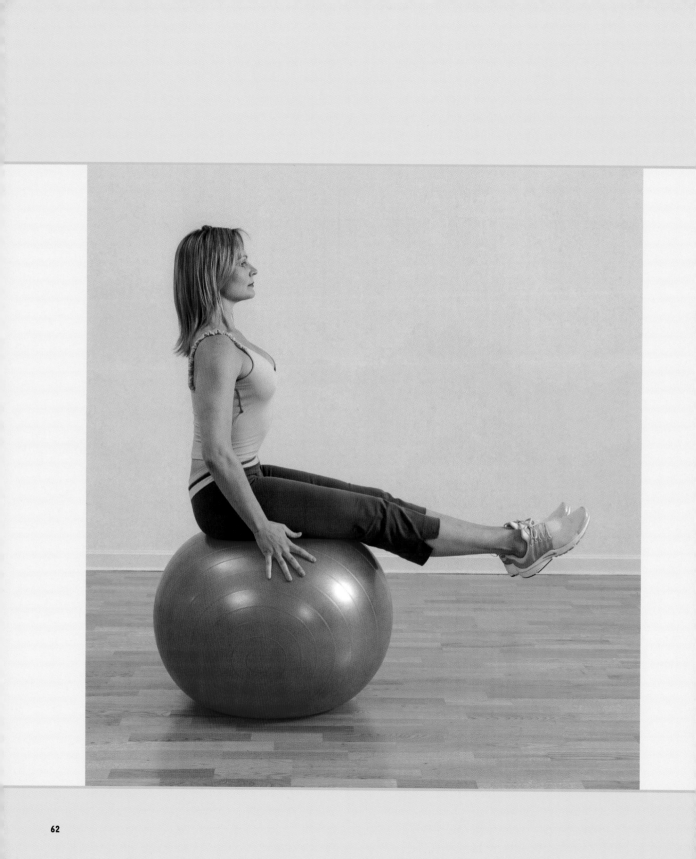

Seated Ball Moves

What could be easier than just sitting on the ball, right? Well, the truth is, sitting on the ball, without rolling, is a difficult exercise in itself. In these moves, you'll not only be sitting, you'll be moving as you sit! It's a lot tougher than it looks and, in fact, people are always surprised at how much trouble they have just sitting on the ball.

It's difficult to sit on the ball because you need to engage your core muscles—your abs and back—in order to remain stable on an unstable surface. When you factor in movement, such as lifting your legs or rolling your arms, then balancing becomes that much more difficult. The most important thing you can do is be sure to keep your powerhouse engaged. This allows you to be in control of your body and thus keep your limbs, as well as your torso, stable.

28 Seated Side Bends

BENEFITS: Lengthens the sides of your body, creating a smaller waist.

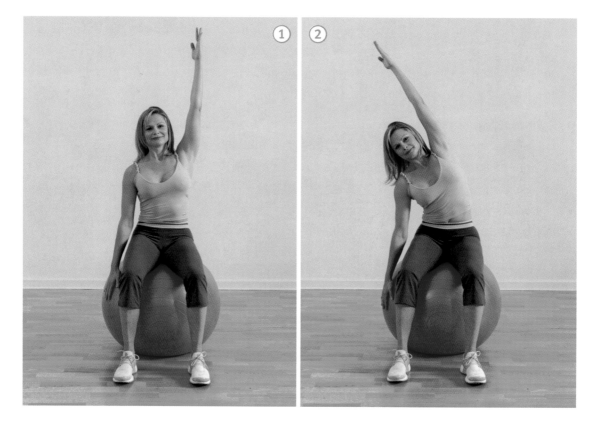

① ②

① Sit on the ball with one arm up, one against the ball.

② Bend to one side, stretching your opposite side long. Be sure not to twist your torso.

③ Return to the center. Alternate sides. Repeat 10-12 times.

29 Seated Leg Extension

BENEFITS: Strengthens your quadriceps muscles.

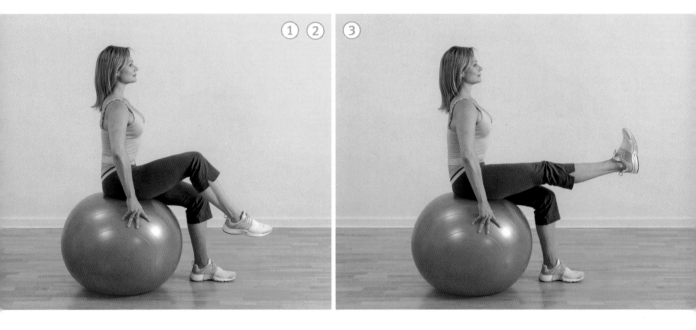

① ② ③

① Sit on the ball. At first, you can hold onto the ball. As you get better at balancing, extend your arms out to the side.

② Lift one knee and straighten your leg, reaching out through your heel.

③ Flex and point your ankle.

④ Return to the starting position. Repeat on the other side. Do this 10-12 times.

30 Seated Knee Crunches

BENEFITS: Strengthens your abs and lower back.

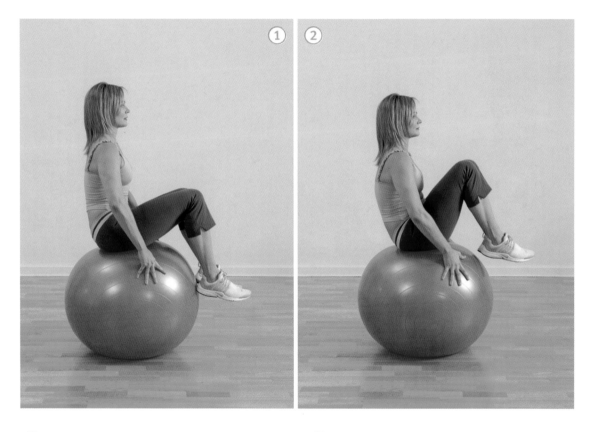

① ②

① Sit on top of the ball with your knees at a right angle to your hips and your hands on the ball.

② Lift both knees at once toward your chest, using your abs to lift your knees.

③ Return back to the starting position. Do this 5 times, working your way up to 15.

31

Seated Hamstring Stretch

BENEFITS: Creates a long, graceful line from your butt to your knee.

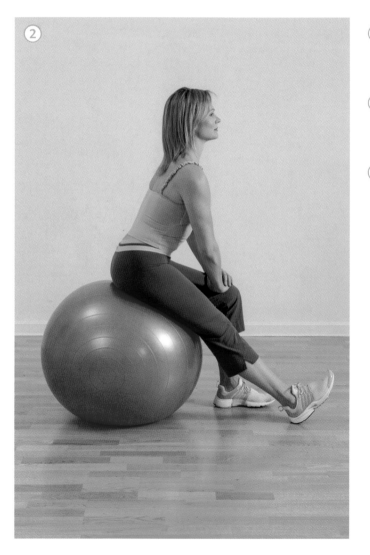

(1) Sit on the ball, one leg extended. Rest your hands on your bent knee.

(2) Bend forward, stretching long through your torso and keeping your butt back.

(3) Change legs. Do this 10-12 times on each leg.

32 Kneeling Side Bend Stretch

BENEFITS: Stretches the sides of your body, opens your chest for more breathing space.

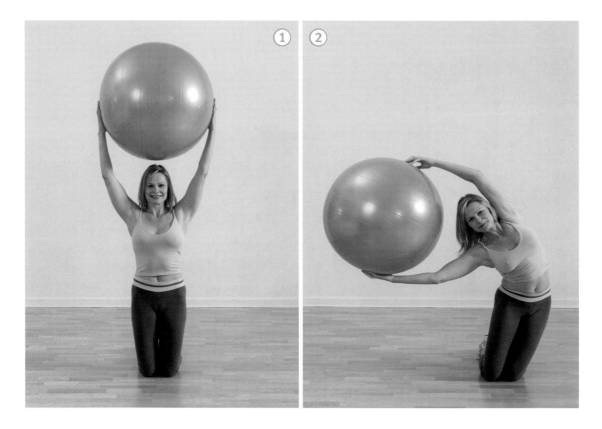

① ②

① Kneel, holding the ball above your head with straight arms.

② Bend to one side with the ball. Your hips should move in the opposite direction. Be sure not to bend forward

at the waist or allow your butt to stick out behind.

③ Come back to center. Do this 5 times to each side.

Standing Ball Slide

BENEFITS: Strengthens and tones leg and butt muscles, as well as the core muscles of the torso. If you keep your arms lifted the whole time, you will also strengthen your triceps and shoulders.

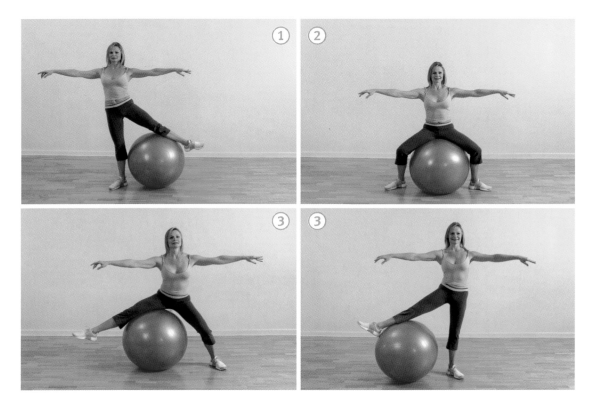

① Stand with the ball between your legs; torso long, and arms to your sides. Keep your shoulders lowered and relaxed. Your left leg should be long over the ball while the weight of your body is in the right leg.

② Come down into a 2nd position plié over the ball.

③ Immediately begin to come back up with your weight on the left leg and the right leg long. Repeat this up to 10 times on each side.

34 Seated Forward Roll

BENEFITS: Stretches your back and upper body, teaches body awareness of your transverse abdominals.

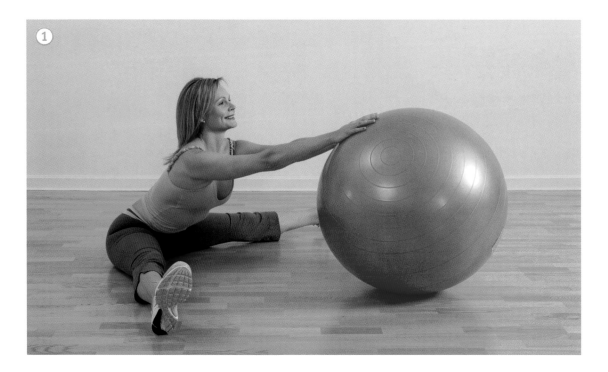

① Sit with your legs in a wide V position, the ball between your thighs.

② Roll the ball forward. Hold the stretch for a few deep breaths.

③ Roll the ball back. Do this 5 times.

35

Extended Forward Roll

BENEFITS: This Pilates move strengthens all of the muscles of the powerhouse—the abs, chest, and upper and lower back.

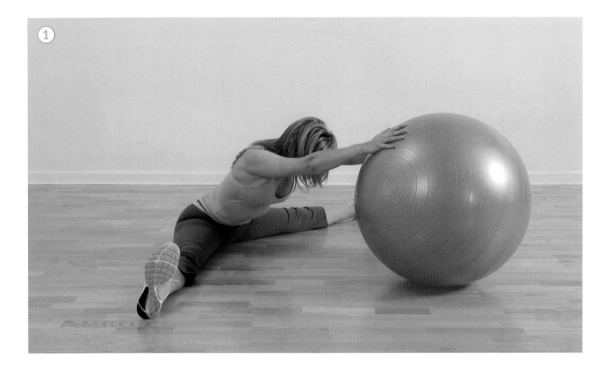

① Sit with your legs a wide V with your hands on top of the ball.

② Roll the ball towards one foot, keeping both hips on floor.

③ Return to the center. Roll the ball to your other foot. Do this 5 times on each side.

Leg Extensions

BENEFITS: Creates long, beautiful legs, like a ballerina.

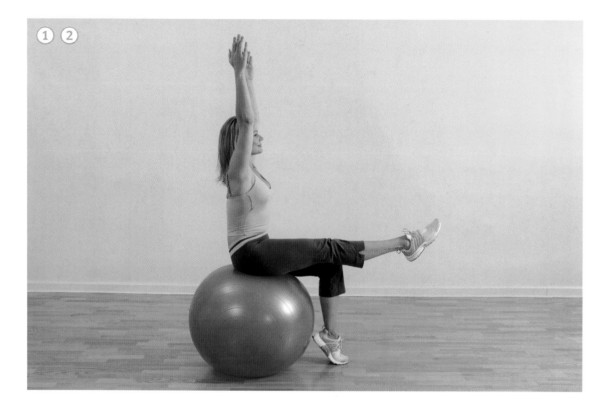

(1)(2)

(1) Sit on the ball, with your knees hip-distance apart, on the balls of your feet. Extend your arms up to the ceiling.

(2) Extend one leg, keeping the heel on the floor raised. Flex and point your lifted, straight leg.

(3) Return to the original position, then repeat with your other leg. Do this 8 times.

Using Weights on the Ball

Using dumbbells as resistance is an important part of any well-rounded exercise program. As we age, our bodies lose muscle mass, which results in weight gain, a loss of strength, and can contribute to losses in mobility and bone density.

Unfortunately, although weight-training is easy and doesn't have to take a lot of time—you only need to do about eight exercises for a whole-body routine—lots of people, especially women, dislike it. I think they find the moves boring and repetitive and they aren't convinced that the results are worth it. Many women believe that lifting weights will make them big, but nothing could be further from the truth. Let me give you a little anatomy lesson, if you don't mind:

When you're young, your muscles are naturally sleek and strong. Sleek and strong muscles keep your skin taut, keep your body lifted, and keep your shape trim and small. As you age and lose your muscle mass, your skin doesn't have a dense enough foundation to rely on, so you develop cellulite. Your body begins to sag because, once again, the upper layers of your body don't have a strong foundation to sit on. And, finally, you get bigger because fat actually takes up more space than muscle. A fat thigh is bigger than a muscular one. Think about a ballet dancer—they're very muscular (really, they're all muscle and no fat) and they aren't big at all.

The fear of getting big is based on the bodies of bodybuilders, whose aim it is get large. They eat to grow and they exercise to grow. But we aren't going to do that. We are only lifting weights to maintain muscle mass, create lean bodies, and improve our posture, skin tone, and overall health.

Lifting weights on the ball is fun and effective. And it's tough! That's because you're working to balance your body as well as move the extra weight you're holding. So, really, it's a great way to work harder without actually lifting a heavier weight than you want to.

Move slowly through any weight routine. Rushing or moving too fast means you're allowing momentum to help with the weight and you want the entire motion to come from the force of your body. Also, focus on form as much as you would during a Pilates or yoga move. When your body is moving properly with dumbbells, you'll feel the move more—and see the results faster.

When I design weight routines for my clients, I always try to incorporate the ball into the exercises. The ball increases the efficacy of any strength move because it forces you to stabilize your core muscles and the joints related to it. Even though we are using weights to strengthen the upper and lower extremities, it's the spine, in relationship to the rib cage and pelvis, that we need to consider to be sure we will properly strengthen our extremities.

In fact, you should begin any exercise or daily activity requiring physical exertion by first thinking about engaging the core muscles properly. We use the core muscles to keep the spine stable because if you don't use your three-dimensional core muscles for proper spinal alignment and support, you won't be able to keep your essential center of gravity and you'll fall off the ball! But, when these core muscles work together with controlled breathing, the trunk is able to easily adjust its supportive response to slight movements and momentum. Meanwhile, the ball's surface assists the superficial muscles to improve the actions of the joints. In fact, the surface of the ball draws attention to your balance; this automatically recruits deep internal core muscles, your navigational system which you may not have been actively (notice I say actively) engaging on your own.

When most people begin weight-lifting, they don't even think about their abs, back, and hips. But this awareness of the importance of your core muscles will quickly become obvious to you and your body will transform itself; your range of motion and balance will be restored, you'll feel more energetic during and after exercise, and your posture will improve. Also, utilizing your core muscles properly will relieve you of any chronic pain caused by muscle imbalances or improper movement patterns.

The best part about all of your hard work? You'll redefine your extremities, sculpting the most symmetrical muscles you've ever had. You'll work deep abdominal layers you didn't know how to properly target, which will give you the flattest abs possible.

You'll need make a conscious effort at first, when sitting or lying on the ball with weights, to connect your front and back trunk muscles prior moving your arms and legs. Ultimately, your core muscles will become like the navigational system you have in your car, directing your breathing, level of energy, and focus.

Always begin with the weights down on the floor until your body has adjusted to the ball and its contouring effects, especially when performing chest and back exercises. The ball adapts to spinal curves, thus recruiting and coordinating smaller structural muscles as a team to stabilize your core. For example, in doing the Shoulder Press, the ball helps you by requiring that you activate your core and lengthen your spine, keep your center of gravity, and stack your hips and shoulders for stability. This becomes even more apparent when you graduate to lifting one foot off floor—your obliques have to work harder to maintain your balance!

The Planes of Your Body

The body has three planes or directions in which it can move: front/back, up/down, and side/side. When a joint is stable in all planes, the muscles that surround it balance and work efficiently. If a joint is not stable, then muscles that are already strong in one plane work first and continue to get stronger, while the weak muscles further deteriorate, which also causes ligaments to overstretch. Remember to concentrate on proper body positioning, because you will be trying to work the muscles that like to stay passive while releasing tension from the muscles screaming to work, because it's more convenient to rely on your existing strength.

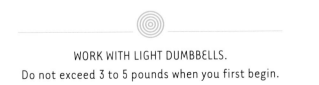

WORK WITH LIGHT DUMBBELLS.
Do not exceed 3 to 5 pounds when you first begin.

37

3-D
Shoulder Press

BENEFITS: This move works the top and front of the shoulders and improves your posture.

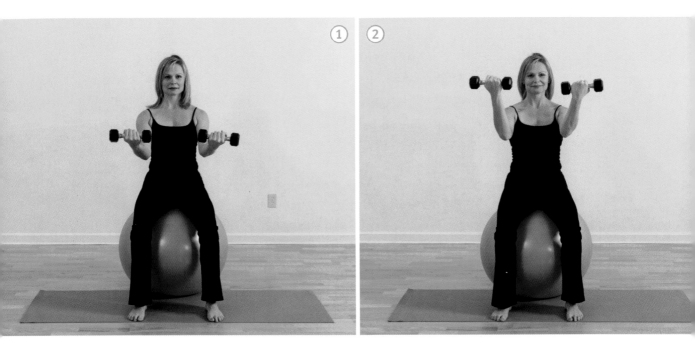

① Sit on top of the ball, feet hip-distance apart, elbows bent and forearms resting on your thighs. Hold a weight in each hand.

② Bring your hands up to shoulder height in a biceps curl. Then, start to raise your arms from the shoulder to come into a shoulder press.

3-D
Shoulder Press

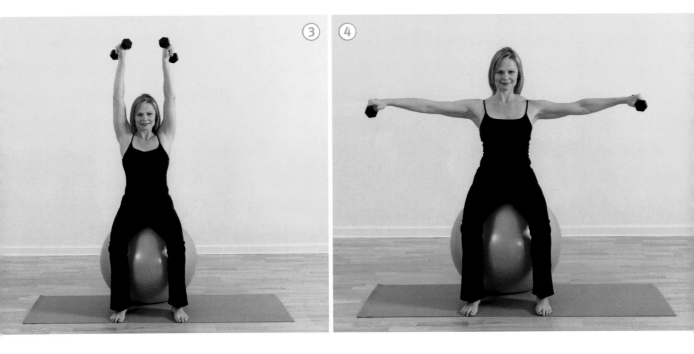

③ Keeping your back stable and your abs contracted, lift your arms up and over your head, turning your palms forward at the top of the shoulder press.

④ Come down slowly. Repeat 4 times.

If you have any problems with your shoulders, modify this exercise by only raising your elbows to nose height and do not straighten your arms. Keep the range of motion small until you build stability in your shoulders.

38 Seated Lateral Raise— One Leg Lifted

BENEFITS: Strengthens and shapes the front of your shoulders while working your powerhouse.

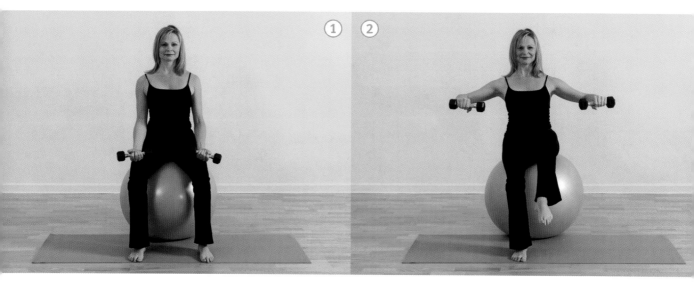

① Sit on top of the ball, feet hip-distance apart, elbows bent and forearms resting on your thighs. Hold a weight in each hand.

② Bring your hands up to shoulder height, raising one leg.

③ Keep one leg raised for 3 reps, then switch legs, either repeating the same arm exercises or reversing the arm movement direction for 3 reps.

④ Come down slowly. Repeat 4 times.

While performing the lift with your knee raised, make sure you engage your obliques and keep your pelvis neutral.

39 Supine Chest Flies

BENEFITS: Strengthens your pectoral (chest) muscles.

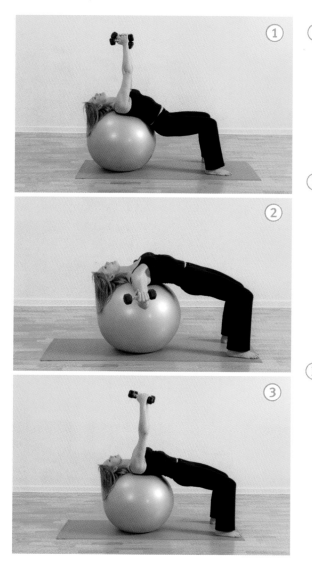

(1) Lie on the ball with your hips lifted into a flat plank position, weights down on the floor alongside your hips. Pick up your weights and bend your elbows to bring the weights alongside your chest. Press your arms up straight, palms facing each other.

(2) Inhale as you open your arms out to the side with your palms facing upward. Initiate the movement with your shoulder blades to stabilize shoulder joint and keep your core strong, maintaining your hips and lower back in the same position throughout the exercise. You will feel a stretch in your chest muscles.

(3) Exhale as you close your arms directly above your chest with palms facing each other. Keep your elbows slightly bent and your wrists in line with your forearm throughout the movement. Do this 8 times. Perform a second set if you wish.

40 Seated Bicep Curls with Single Leg Lift

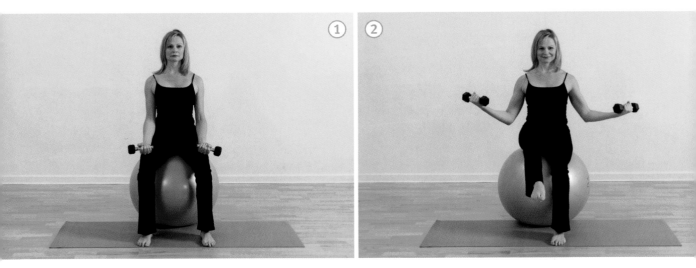

① ②

① Sit on top of the ball with your elbows at hip-level, holding the weights palm up with a loose grip. Engage your core muscles three-dimensionally to establish proper shoulder alignment.

② Lift one foot about six inches from floor with a relaxed thigh to target your oblique abdominals and deep core supporting muscles on each side.

③ Curl your hands up to your shoulder and then lower them back down. Repeat 8 times. Lower your leg and lift the opposite leg. Repeat the curl 8 times.

Try to keep your hips aligned to insure the correct muscles are firing in your core. Take a mindful approach to feel the relationship between your ribs, arms, and pelvis, and try to keep them in alignment. This will keep your shoulders aligned as well.

41

Single Arm Chest Reach Across

BENEFITS: A creative way to lift and strengthen your pectoral muscles.

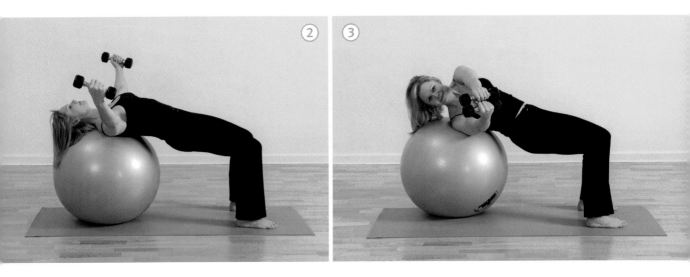

② ③

① Lie on the ball in an incline bench press position, with your hips lifted into plank position, weights on the floor alongside your hips to begin. Pick up your weights and bend your elbows to bring the weights alongside your chest.

② Open your arms straight out to the side, slightly higher than your trunk, initiating the movement by pressing your shoulder blades into the ball to stabilize your shoulder joint.

③ Move one arm across to meet the other, with the ultimate goal of getting both palms to meet. Follow the weight with your eyes throughout the movement. Alternate 4 times to each side.

◎

Keep your hips steadily aligned, knees directly in line with your hips, ankles below knees, with your weight evenly distributed between your heels and toes. This will stretch and strengthen the deep layers of your core.

Seated Front and Lateral Bicep Curls, One Leg Raised

BENEFITS: Strengthens and tones the front of your upper arms while flatting your abdominal muscles.

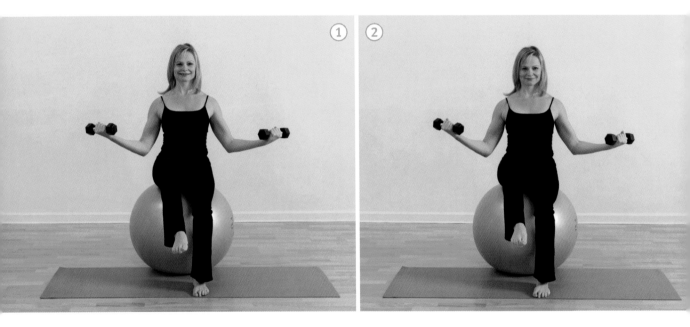

(1) Sit on top of the ball, elbows bent even with your hips, holding a weight in each hand, and one foot lifted a few inches off the floor.

(2) Bend your elbows into a bicep curl.

(3) Lower the weights through a full range motion down to the ball.

(4) Bend your elbows, rotating your arms out. Do this 10 times.

43

Decline Bicep Curls over Ball

BENEFITS: A concentrated way to define your upper arms.

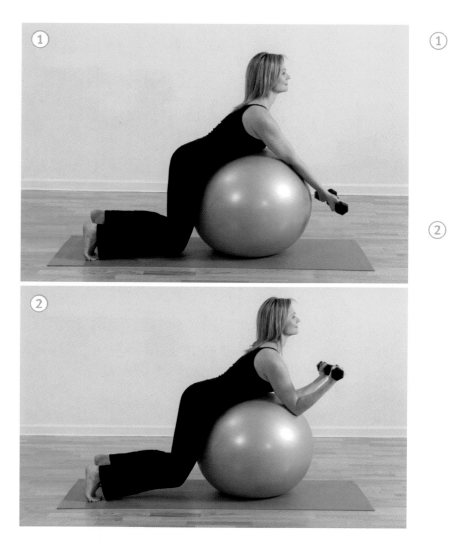

1. Kneel on the floor with your chest on the ball, thighs against the ball, on the balls of your feet. Extend your arms, holding weights, straight, palms up.

2. Curl your palms up to your shoulder and then lower them back down. Firmly press elbows into the ball. Do this 10 times.

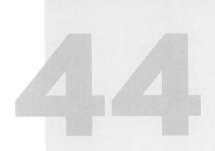

Side Lying Fly

BENEFITS: This move isolates your pectoral muscles, giving lift to your bust.

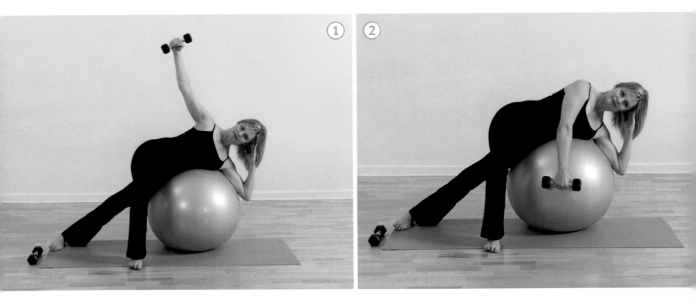

(1) Lie with your left side on the ball, left leg extended straight and right leg crossed over it, knee bent. Support your head with your left hand (elbow bent). Your arms are open in fly position with weights.

(2) One arm closes to the center of your chest, your trunk stays straight.

(3) Return to starting position. Do this 10 times on each side.

45

Decline
Bench Press

BENEFITS: Strengthens your chest and shoulder muscles.

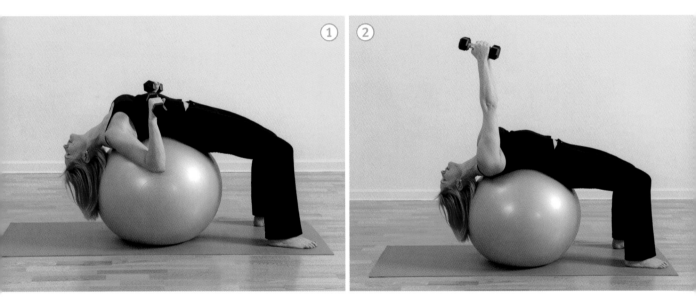

① Lie over the ball with your head and shoulders back over the ball in the decline position. Your arms should assume a bench press position, with your elbows bent into the ball and your palms facing forward.

② Straighten both arms while keeping them in line with your chest. Squeeze your shoulders down while turning your palms to face each other.

③ Return your elbows back to the ball. Do this 10 times.

46

Overhead Triceps Press

BENEFITS: Strengthens and tones the back of the upper arm.

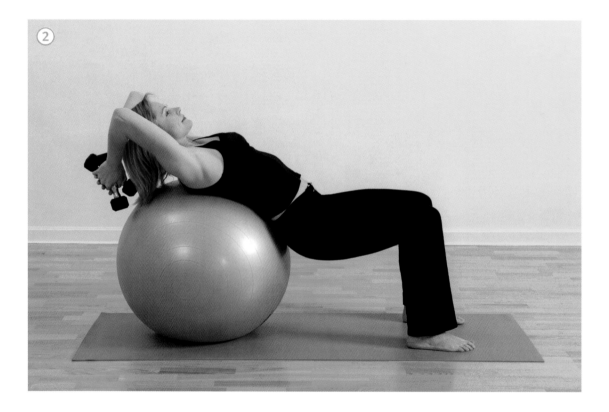

① Lie on your back on the ball in the incline position. Hold the weights with your elbows bent back overhead. Keep the back of your shoulders pressed into the ball with your elbows pressed in.

② Extend your arms out straight, without moving your elbows.

③ Return to start position. Do this 10 times.

47

Side Bend on Ball with Weights

BENEFITS: Strengthens and shapes the front of your shoulder muscle.

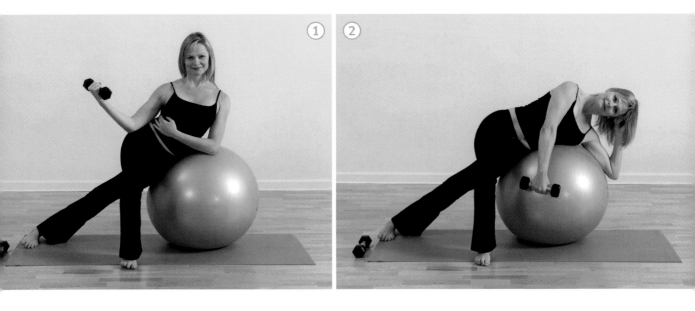

① Lie on your side; stretch and contour the side of your body over the ball. Your hip should be against the ball and your bottom leg extended straight, top leg crosses over and foot rests on the floor. Wrap your bottom arm around your ribs; your top arm holds the weight, elbow on top of your pelvis.

② Lean further down on the ball, supporting your head with your hand, and rotate your hand and forearm down towards the floor until your arm is straight.

③ Return elbow back to hip position. Do this 10-12 times.

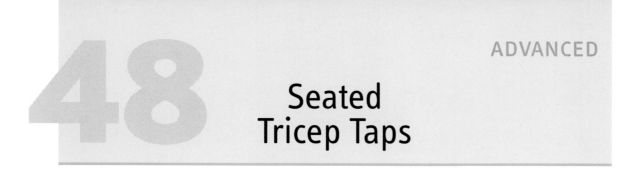

48

Seated
Tricep Taps

BENEFITS: Tones the back of your upper arms.

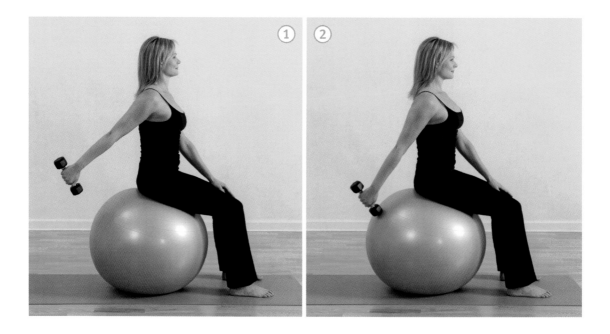

(1) Sit on the ball with your arm extended behind your hip, palm facing in.

(2) Lift the weight up off ball.

(3) Lower your arm, tapping the weight down with your elbow straight. Do this 10 times with each arm.

49

Prone Upper
Back Rows

BENEFITS: Strengthens the upper and middle portions of your back, improves your posture.

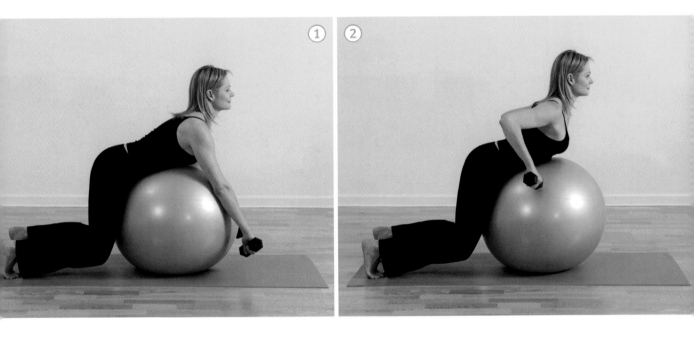

① On your knees, drape your chest over the ball with your hips pressed firmly into the ball. Pick up your weights, with your palms face in and your arms straight in front of the ball.

② Pull your shoulder blades together, opening your chest. Bend your elbows back and lift them to the ceiling, pressing your rib cage into the ball.

③ Return to the stretch position. Do this 10 times.

50 Lateral Shoulder Raises, One Leg Raised

BENEFITS: Strengthens the middle of your shoulders and tightens your abdominal muscles.

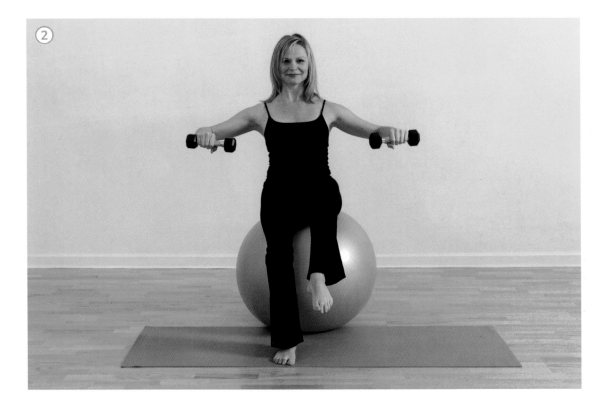

1. Sit on the ball, your elbows bent to your sides and your hands forward. One foot should be off the floor.

2. Raise your elbows out and up to shoulder height.

3. Lower your elbows. Repeat 6 times then change legs. Do another 6 lifts.

51 Side Bends with Weight and Straight Leg

BENEFITS: This is a great, creative way to work your back and oblique muscles. You also have to keep your ab muscles engaged in order to stay on the ball. It's tough!

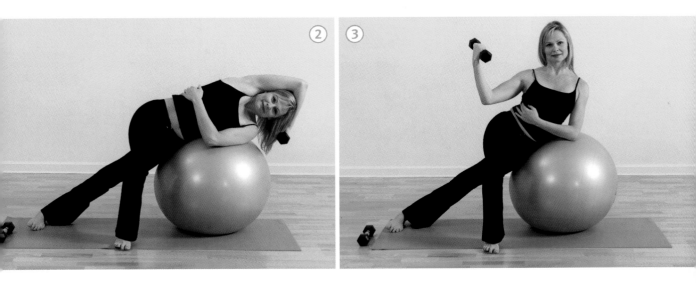

1. Lay on one side, stretching your side body over ball, hip against the ball, with your bottom leg extended straight and your top leg crossed over it, foot on the floor.

2. Wrap your bottom arm around your waist while your top arm, holding a dumbbell, comes up over your head. Hold the weight gently without flexing at the wrist.

3. Inhale and pull your top ribs and hip together as you lift your torso up off the ball. Your arm will move with your body and come into a flexed position at the elbow. Be sure your neck is relaxed and your shoulders are down. Hold for one or two seconds in the contraction. Make sure you keep your torso in alignment as you move.

4. Return back to the stretch position. Do up to 10 times, then repeat on the other side.

52 Prone Tricep Extensions

BENEFITS: Tones the back of your upper arms.

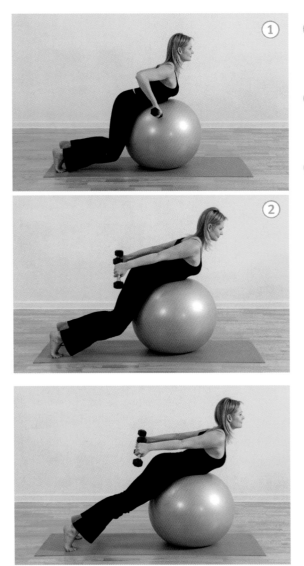

① Lie prone with full trunk over ball, legs wide and slightly bent. Bend your elbows up to point to the ceiling.

② Straighten your arms with a twisting action of the upper arm, pinky finger rotating in.

③ Return to bent elbows. Repeat 10 times.

You can turn this into a back extension as well if you straighten your legs and pull your arms back without clenching your shoulders together.

53 Decline Chest Press

BENEFITS: Adds lift to your chest.

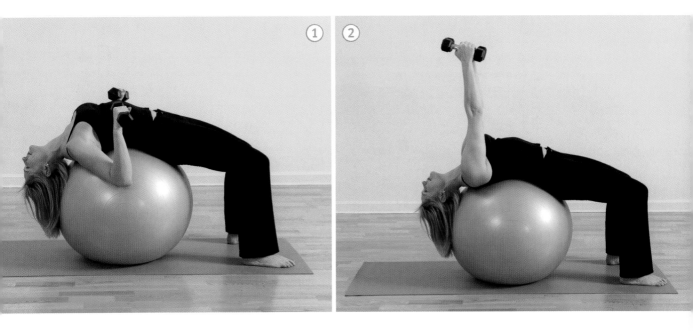

(1) (2)

(1) Lie with your back on the ball, neck stretched and head back, weights in your hands above your chest. Your head should be back on ball.

(2) Open your arms wide with slightly bent elbows.

(3) Raise and close your arms, palms face in. Then return to start. Do this 10-12 times.

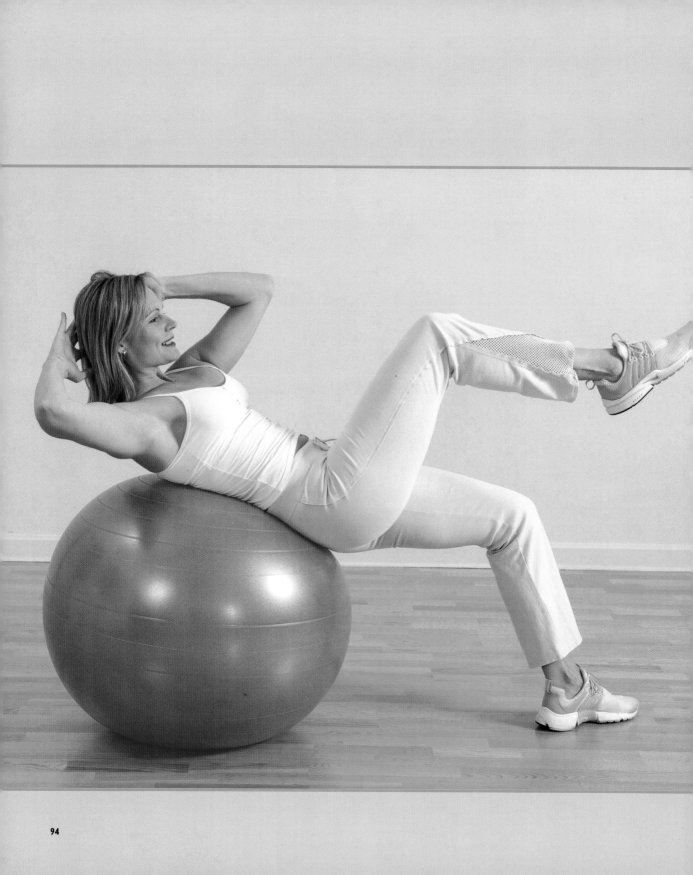

Supine Moves
with the Ball

These abdominal exercises are favorites of my clients. The ball is so effective as a prop for ab work because of its shape and surface. The ball contours to your spine so you have an easier time maintaining your form when exercising on your own than if you were on the floor. It places your spine into its natural lumbar, and cervical curvature alignment. So, instead of lying on a hard wooden floor to do crunches, your body will instead be in a neutral position, allowing your abs to do all of the work. You'll have to do fewer reps and you'll see faster, better results.

There are two positions to address before getting started:

1. **Supine or flat on floor with knees over ball:** You can place the ball against a wall for some of the exercises if you require extra support when just starting out.

2. **Supine on top of the ball:** It's best to sit on the ball first when starting off and then move down to adjust the stretch. Make sure your ribs are actively stretching away from your pelvis, with your tailbone resting gently into the ball.

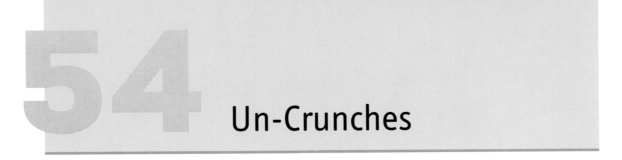

54 Un-Crunches

BENEFITS: This is the best way to learn how to properly do a crunch, because the point of this exercise isn't to "crunch" your muscles, but to create long, flat abs.

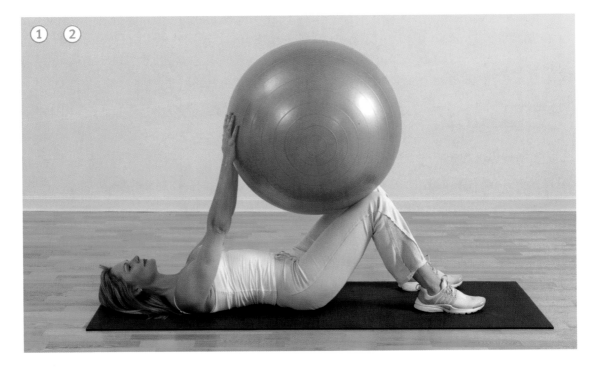

① ②

① Lie on your back, knees bent, feet flat on the floor. Place the ball between your hands and knees. Keep your arms straight.

② Begin by first moving the ball back and forth gently between your hands and knees. Keep your spine long, and your skull on the floor without arching your neck or lower back. This placement activates your core.

Un-Crunches

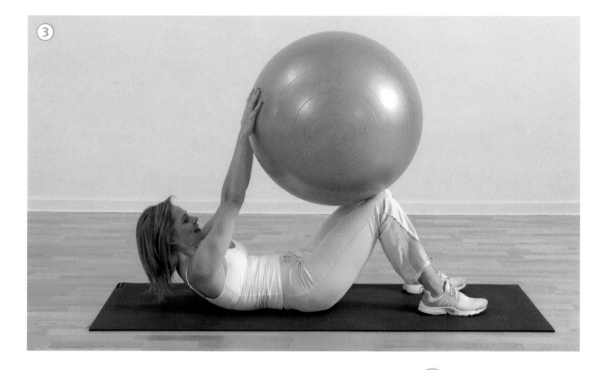

(3) Raise your head, neck, and shoulders off the floor, without pressing too hard with your hands. The spine should remain stable on the ground, without arching. Keep your tailbone firmly on the floor. Repeat this 8-10 times.

Your hands should be placed in front of the ball, shoulder's width apart, your palms totally flat on top. Your elbows must be straight at all times or else your fulcrum will change. This is very important to remember, because if your arms bend at the elbow joint, the kinesthetic chain of energy flow has changed. You will have lost the assistance of the scapula to move the leverage forwards. This action is important to counterbalance the force the knees are applying to the arms and vice versa.

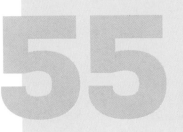

Floor Criss-Cross

BENEFITS: Strengthens and tones the oblique muscles, creating a lean torso and smaller waist.

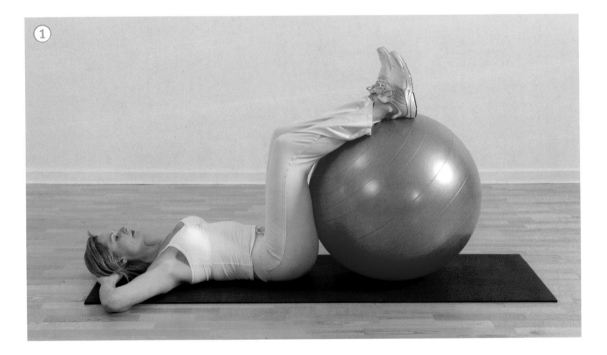

① Lie on your back on the floor, elbows bent with your hands placed behind your head. Your knees should be bent over the ball with your feet loose. Your spine is long between your ribs and pelvis, and your tailbone must remain pressed into the floor.

② Use your bent knees to pull the ball close into your buttocks, and use your hamstrings to secure the neutral pelvis position, tailbone pointed towards the ball.

Floor Criss-Cross

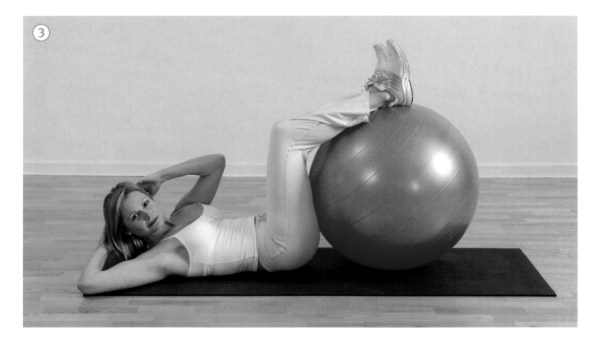

③ After you have established the locked position of the pelvis, keep the ball still while you begin crossing one elbow towards your opposite knee. You should have a mental image of making a long diagonal line from your shoulder to your opposite hip. Press your opposite elbow into the ground. Do not do a downward crunch, which would prevent your obliques from doing the major part of the work.

④ Return to a neutral flat position. Alternate sides. Do 5 times on each side. Perform up to two sets.

◎

Your oblique abdominals are deeper and typically weaker than your other abdominal muscles. Plus, one side is usually stronger than the other. This is especially true in scoliosis patients and people who sit for long periods. Focus on the side that feels weaker in order to create more balance in your body.

56 Reverse Crunch on Floor

BENEFITS: Strengthens your core muscles, specifically the lower portion of your rectus abdominal muscle.

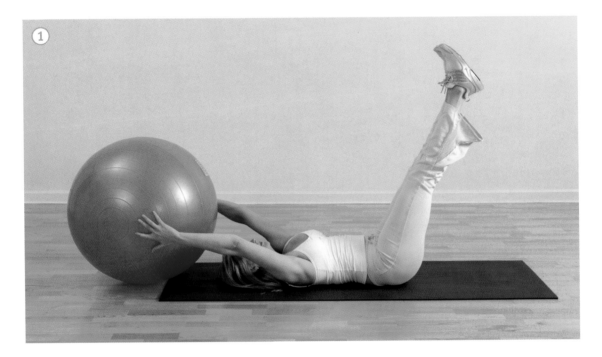

① Lie on your back on the floor. Place the ball on the floor overhead, holding it on either side, with your arms about twelve inches off floor, so your shoulder girdle is stable and your lats are stretched to prepare core leverage. Your legs point up to the ceiling, as straight as possible. Begin by pulling your thigh bones together and into your hip sockets. Think only of your bones working to lock your joints, instead of your muscles which can over-tighten or hyper-extend, hindering your balance. Hold your legs firmly together in a parallel position by lining up your ankle joints, the insides of your knees, and your upper thigh bones.

Reverse Crunch on Floor

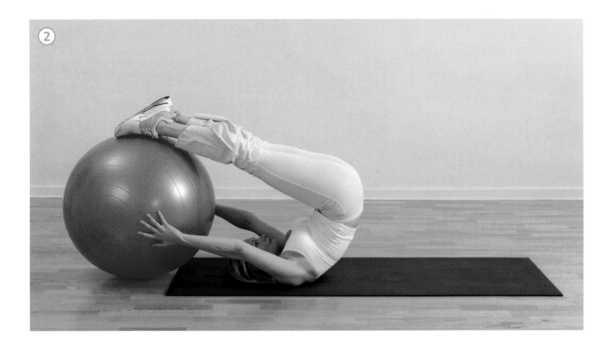

② Lower your legs halfway to the ground, with your core engaged to brace your center. Feel your abs begin to stretch as you continue to pull your navel down to the ground. Don't let your lower back leave the floor! At the point where you feel your muscular control is about to run out, roll your legs overhead, exhaling into the muscles surrounding your rib cage. Your feet end up resting on top of the ball with a flat line from your sit bones to your heels.

③ Exhale and roll down vertebra by vertebra, using the ball to brace your upper body. Repeat 4-6 times.

If your neck or lower back feel any strain, leave this exercise out until you develop strength, or modify it by not dropping your legs too far down towards the floor or all the way over your head. Go only as far as you feel comfortable, increasing the range of motion when your strength and flexibility improve.

Teaser with Twist

BENEFITS: Increases your spinal flexibility and strengthens core muscles.

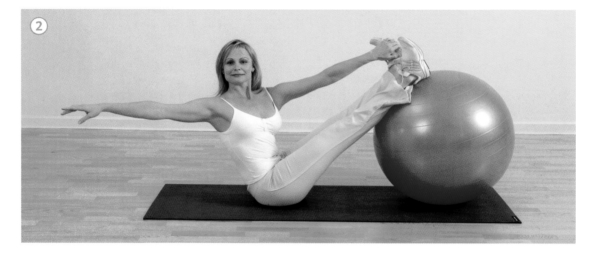

① Lie on your back on the floor. Bend your knees, into a right angle position with your heels parallel and resting on top of the ball, your arms reaching straight over your head.

② Inhale and reach your arms off the floor, towards the ball, at the same time rolling the ball forward with your heels. Your trunk should follow the ball as it rolls, imitating the movement quality of the ball, without over-contracting your midsection. As your spine reaches its straightest possible position, without over-tightening the muscles on top of your thighs, reach your arms into

a twisting letter T. Bend your knees if your back is sinking.

③ Return your arms back to the center, reaching straight forward, and roll back down evenly through each vertebra of the spine. Gradually bend your knees to the starting position, returning your arms back overhead. Repeat 5 times.

Keep your knees slightly bent if your hamstrings are tight. If your body is not floating up off the floor, then remind yourself to relax the larger superficial "crunch" muscle layer.

58

Supine Ball Wall Roll

BENEFITS: Strengthens the hamstrings and the entire powerhouse.

(1) Lie on your back with the ball close to a wall and your feet on the ball, back flat against the floor.

(2) Roll the ball up and down the wall by bending your knees and lifting your hips. You'll have to really press the ball with your feet. Try to keep your shoulders relaxed and don't clench the floor with your hands. Feel the move in your hips and pelvis.

(3) Pay special attention to the alignment of your hips, knees, and feet. They should remain parallel at hip-width apart. Repeat 5 times.

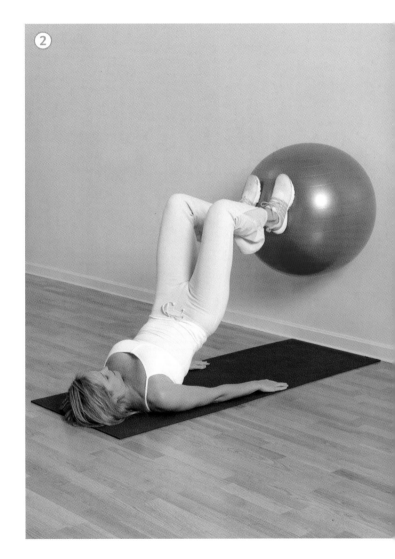

59 Supine Hip Hammock Swing

BENEFITS: Strengthens the muscles of your thighs and hips.

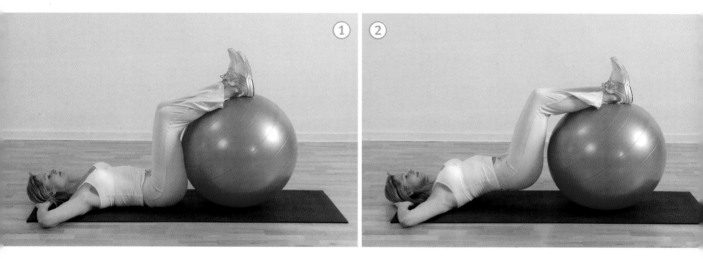

① Lie on your back on the floor, your knees bent at a right angle over the ball. Press your thighs firmly together and the crease line of your knees into the top of the ball. Keep your feet in as much of a neutral ankle position as possible.

② Begin by simultaneously engaging your abs and your hip muscles, pulling the bones of your legs together and lifting your hips off the floor with a soft, swinging forward motion.

③ Return your hips back to the floor, pulling the ball back into the back of your legs. Use a swinging, controlled downward motion, keeping the muscles in your front and back thighs working. Do this 10 times. Add another set if you wish.

Try not to straighten your knees or over-extend your ankles while rolling the ball. Maintaining a neutral ankle placement will help you to keep your hamstrings active when your feet are on the ball.

60

Walking Spinal Roll

BENEFITS: Stretches your back and strengthens your abs and quadriceps. Eases tension in your upper body.

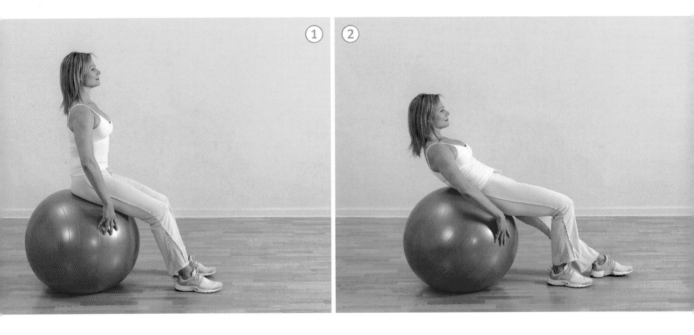

① Sit on the ball with your hips just below the top of the ball.

② With your hands on the ball, walk your feet forward one step at a time until your body is lying back on the ball.

③ Walk back to a sitting position. Repeat 2 to 5 times.

61

Supine Pelvic Press Up

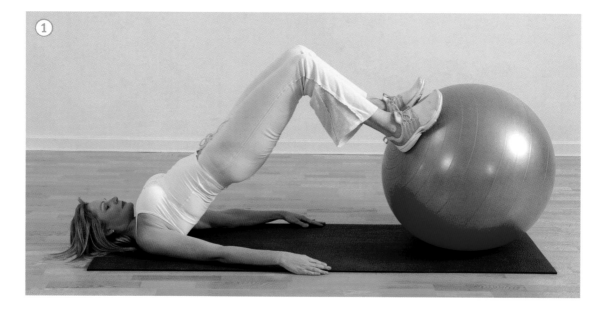

1. Lie on your back on the floor with your knees bent at a right angle, your feet firmly planted into the ball with your heels and all ten toes evenly weighted on the ball. Your thighs are parallel, with your second toe lining up with your knee cap.

2. Maintain a neutral spine. Engage your thigh muscles from the sides and back to brace your weight into the ball, then inhale to prepare, and exhale from your pelvic floor as you connect your deep core muscles with your thighs to lift your hips off the floor. Raise your trunk up until you're on your shoulder blades. Make your spine an extended and level support, connecting your pelvis and rib cage together in a flat line. Lift your hips up and down 10 times, then add a holding pulse up for 10 counts.

Think of pulling the ball closer towards your body instead of pushing it away from you. Pushing against the ball makes you work too much from the front of your thighs, instead of using the pulling action of your hamstrings.

62 Hamstring Roll

BENEFITS: Strengthens the hamstrings.

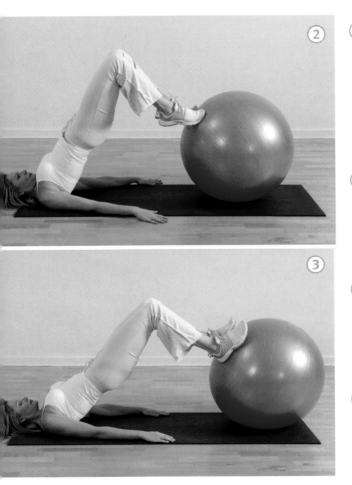

(1) Lie on your back on the floor with your knees bent at a right angle, your feet firmly planted into the ball with your heels and all ten toes evenly weighted on the ball. Your thighs are parallel, with your second toe lining up with your knee cap.

(2) Lift your hips up, roll onto your toes, your heels off the ball, rolling the ball inwards towards your buttocks, while your pelvis lifts as high up on top of your toes as possible.

(3) Lower your heels back to the ball, and lower down to floor. Keep the action slow and your thighs actively working to support your trunk. You will really feel your hamstrings with this one!

(4) Remember to maintain a neutral spinal position and exhale when lifting off, initiating the move from your lifted pelvic floor. Do this 10 times.

63

Diamond Hip Lifts

BENEFITS: This move strengthens your abdominal, inner thigh, and butt muscles.

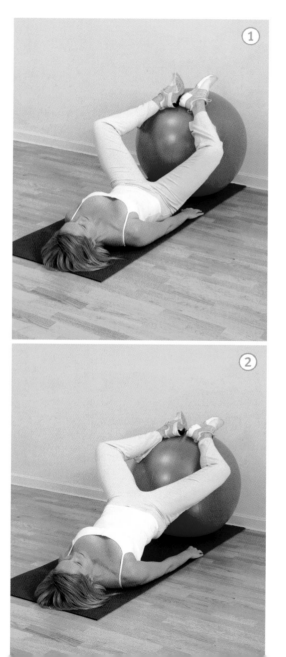

① To help keep the ball steady, you can place it against the wall (optional). Lie on your back on the floor, with your legs on top of the ball and the soles of your feet together, knees open out to the side. Apply pressure to the ball with the outside of your feet, on the pinky toe side, and continue pressing your knees open wide, recruiting the back of your hips, while stretching your inner thighs.

② Lift your hips up and down off the floor, maintaining a diamond shape in between your thighs. Keep the front of your pelvis open and flat. Repeat the exercise 10 times, and then hold your hips up, pulsing for 10.

If you're tight in your inner thighs, it's best to use this exercise initially as a stretch, remaining in the position on the floor. When you are ready to lift, think of your body moving up and down in one piece, pressing weight into your feet.

64 Supine Alternate Straight Leg Lifts

BENEFITS: This is one of my favorite moves to tone and lengthen the entire leg, like a dancer's! Concentrate on your bottom leg and you'll really feel the toning of your butt.

① Lie on your back on the floor, your knees bent at a right angle over the ball so your feet are actually over the other side of ball. Press your thighs firmly together and the crease line of your knees into the top of the ball. Your feet should remain together and softly pointed, getting ready for action!

② Lift up both hips until your weight is on your shoulder blades. Press the back of your lower legs into the ball to support your back, and engage your thighs from behind with your buttocks.

③ Raise one leg until it is at a right angle with your hips. Extend out through the toes of both legs. Keep your hips and the muscles of the bottom leg engaged to maintain the straight line of your body from your shoulders to your toes. Lower the leg. Switch legs. Alternate lifting your legs 8 times (4 on each leg). You can come down between lifts to readjust your position on the ball and rest. Make this exercise easier by keeping both knees bent.

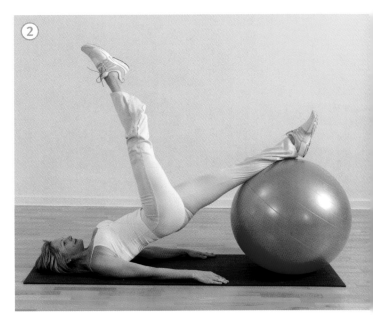

Keep both hips perfectly straight across. Press one leg up, keeping a ninety-degree angle between your thigh and hip, then straighten your knee—that's a much better full range hamstring stretch for stability. Most people tend to take their knee back toward their chest initially, instead of up, but this is not very good for your back.

101 Ways to Work Out on the Ball   **109**

65 Supine Hamstring Stretch

BENEFITS: Stretches and relaxes the back of your leg.

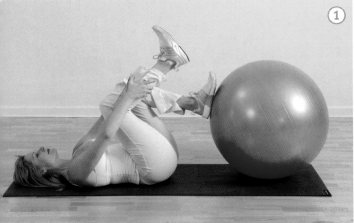 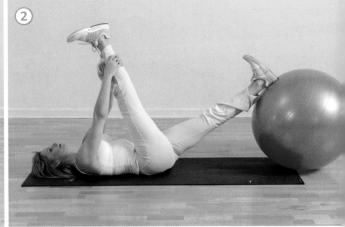

① Lie on your back on the floor, with your knees bent at a right angle and both feet flat on the ball. Bring one leg toward your chest and hold it with both hands—behind your knee if you're less flexible, closer to your ankle if you're very flexible.

If you need to, modify this stretch by bending your legs. This is a favorite stretch of mine. I suggest doing a stretch like this several times a day, even without a ball, especially after doing any cardiovascular exercise or sport.

---

② Begin to straighten both legs simultaneously. Extend the leg you're holding up, using your hands behind either your calf or knee to help support the stretch. The other leg rolls the ball forward to help release the tension out of your hip flexors and psoas muscles, while assisting in maintaining the neutral pelvis position.

③ Return the ball, actively pulling your thigh bones down into your hip sockets while your tailbone pulls deeper away from your body towards floor. Keep a neutral position in your pelvis. Switch legs. Do 5 times on each leg.

66

Inner Thigh
Twists

BENEFITS: Tones your inner and outer thigh muscles, as well as your abdominals.

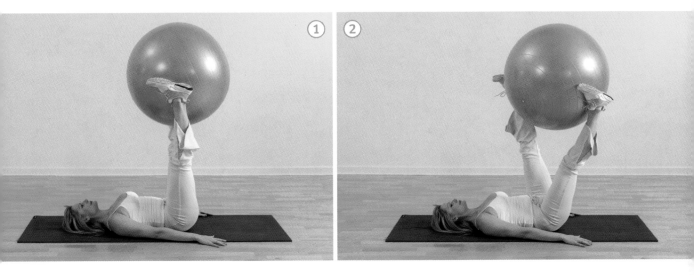

① Lie on your back on the floor. Place the ball between your legs, keeping your legs as straight as possible. Your lower back should remain flat on the floor, and your neck long. If your back is coming off the floor, place a towel or mat under the lowest section of your lumbar spine (the very base of your back). Squeeze the ball tightly with your side and back thighs, turning your inner thighs out slightly from your hip.

② Use your core to stabilize your spine on the floor and begin twisting the ball, using your inner thighs to initiate the twist, while your back and side thigh muscles act with a pulling motion, moving your thigh bones deeper downward into their sockets. This will keep your pelvis neutral and work your hips dynamically in all planes. Repeat 8 times continuously moving and twisting deeper through each repetition.

67

Tricep Dips

BENEFITS: A test of balance, core strength, stability, and upper body strength.

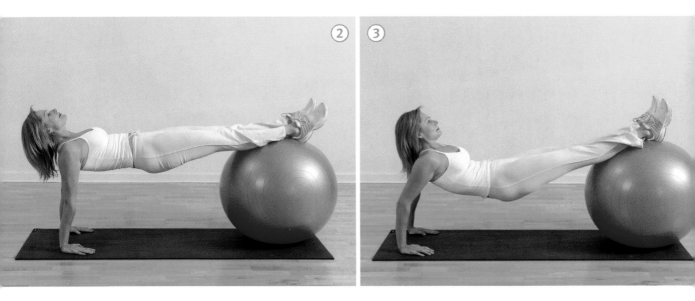

① Begin seated, facing the ball, with your hands behind your back. Place your hands under your shoulders, fingertips pointing toward your rear. Your elbows will move straight back; keep them lined up with your shoulders. This will help stabilize your shoulder joint, so your weight isn't just in your arms. Move your legs so they are flat across the top of the ball in a parallel position.

② Lift your hips off of the floor so that your legs, torso, and head are all in one line. This is very hard, and tests your control of your trunk muscles.

Tricep Dips

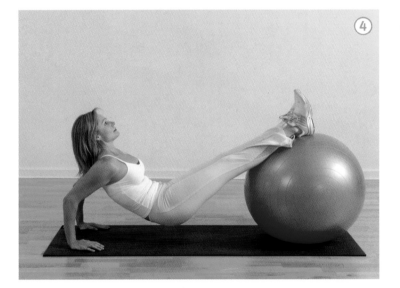

④

Keep your midsection lifted at
all times to avoid dropping
into your shoulders.
Bring your legs further
up onto the ball to
assist the movement.

③ Begin to lower your body, bending your
elbows while allowing them to move
back. Try to shift your weight up off
your arms with your hips. Engage your
abdominal muscles to help support the
weight of your trunk off of your shoulder joints.

④ Lower until you feel your shoulders
beginning to lose stability or your
middle sagging. Stretch your arms
and lift back to the beginning posture.
Repeat up to ten times. For a super
challenge: Add a second set or lift one
leg while doing your reps.

C-Curve Scoop

BENEFITS: This is a basic move for creating a flat front torso and the proper curve in your lower spine.

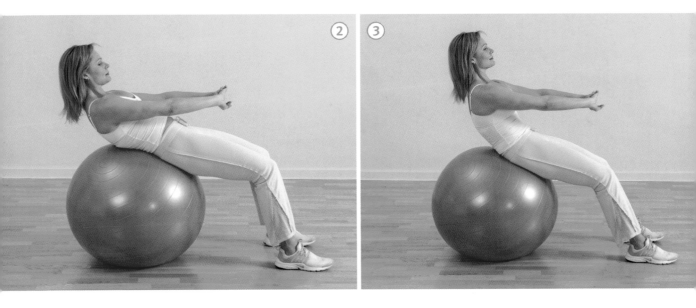

(1) Begin by sitting on the ball, sit slightly in front of the top of the ball, towards your feet.

(2) Roll the ball forwards, lowering your lower and middle back onto the ball, keeping your upper back rounded. Contour your trunk into the curves of your ball.

(3) Straighten your arms out in front of you, and scoop up your abs, lifting your middle back off the ball. Think of pressing the lower back into the ball, instead of lifting away from it, and elongating your trunk instead of over-crunching in the middle. Exhale as you move your arms up and your waist back. Repeat 10 times.

69

Rolling Bridge on Toes

BENEFITS: Relaxes and stretches your hip flexors and quadriceps while strengthening your glutes and hamstrings.

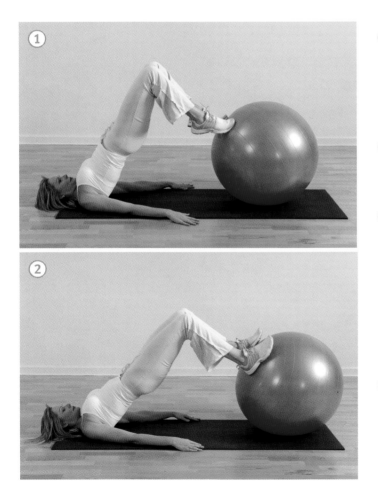

(1) Lie on your back, feet on the ball, hip-distance apart. Lift your hips slightly while pressing your toes into the ball.

(2) Lift your hips further as you roll the ball out, pressing your feet into the ball.

(3) Continue to lift your hips, pressing gently into your shoulders and upper back without crunching your neck. Hold for a few seconds. For an extra challenge, come up all the way onto your toes.

(4) Lower your back slowly to the floor. Repeat 5 times.

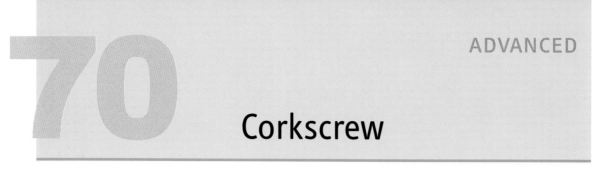

Corkscrew

BENEFITS: Increases core strength and stretches the back and hamstrings, as well as the shoulders.

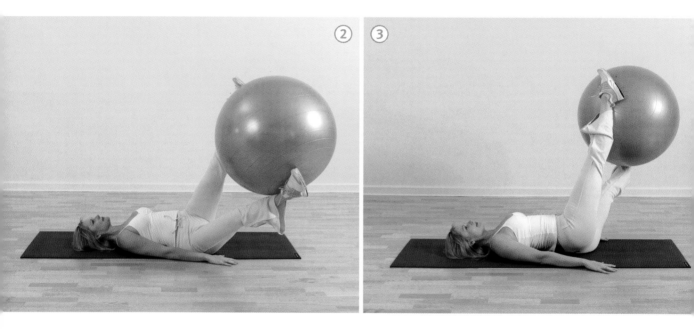

① Lie on your back with your legs stretched straight, ball between your feet. Keep your arms long by your sides and head, shoulders, and neck pressed gently to the floor.

② Lift your hips up, holding the ball with your feet, as you pull your legs and the ball up and over your head. Try not to clench the floor with your hands.

③ Without moving your shoulders, move your hips in a corkscrew or figure-8 shape, lifting as high as you can comfortably onto your shoulders.

④ Come down slowly, lowering each vertebra one at a time to the floor. Repeat 2-5 times.

71

Supine Ball Wall Roll

BENEFITS: This is a fun exercise, but it's tough, too! You'll really need to engage your core muscles to keep the ball—and your body—steady!

(1) Lie on the floor, both feet firmly pressing into the ball.

(2) Roll the ball up the wall as your body rolls up off floor, one vertebra at a time, until your weight is on your shoulders. If that hurts your neck, don't roll up so far.

(3) Roll ball and back down. Repeat 2 times, working your way up to 5 times.

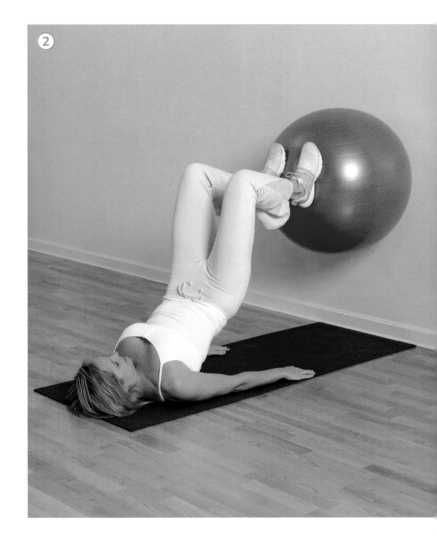

72

Uncrunches on the Ball

BENEFITS: Creates a strong powerhouse and a flat front torso.

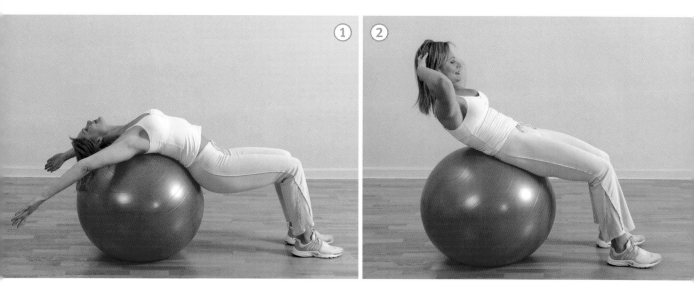

① ②

① Lie with your back on the ball, arms strretched out behind you. Bring your hands behind your head, elbows out to the sides.

② Come up to straight back position, keeping your abs contracted.

③ Release to the start position. Do this 5 times, working your way up to 10.

73

Ball Hip
Rotator Stretch

BENEFITS: Stretches your gluteus and hips.

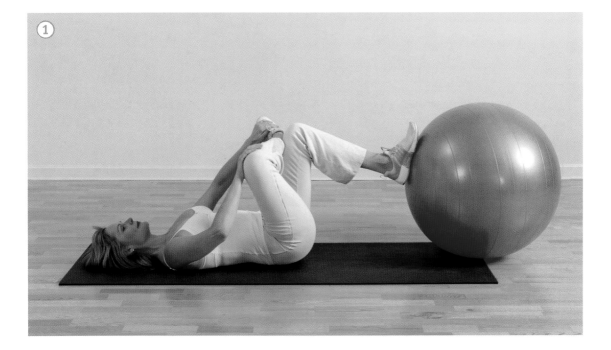

① Lie on your back with one foot on the ball and the opposite leg's ankle crossed onto your knee.

② Roll the ball toward your body, pressing the knee of your crossed-over leg open. Return to the starting position, and repeat up to 10 times.

ADVANCED

Pelvic Lifts

BENEFITS: Strengthens your inner groin and pelvic floor muscles (these are great if you've recently had kids!).

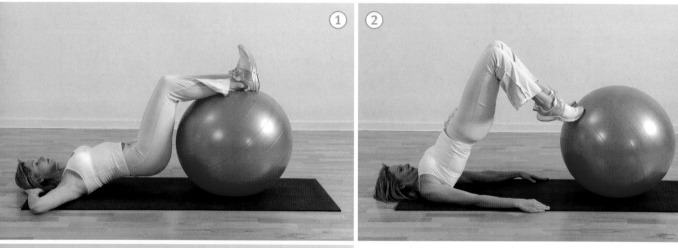

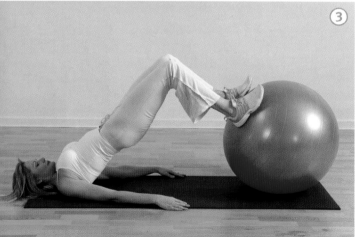

① Lie on the floor with your knees bent at a right angle. Your feet should be on the ball.

② Lift your hips off the floor using your hamstrings and butt.

③ Bring your hips back down all the way, working your legs and butt both ways. Do this 5 times, working your way up to 10.

Backbend Balance

BENEFIT: What a great stretch for your front torso! Increases flexibility in your spine, too, while also strengthening your hip flexors.

1. Sit on the ball and contour your body into the ball while rolling into a backbend position, hands back on the floor.

2. Lift both legs up as much as possible. If you can't balance, lift one leg up at a time.

3. Drop one leg back down at a time and roll up slowly, hands behind your head. Do 1 time and no more than 2 times.

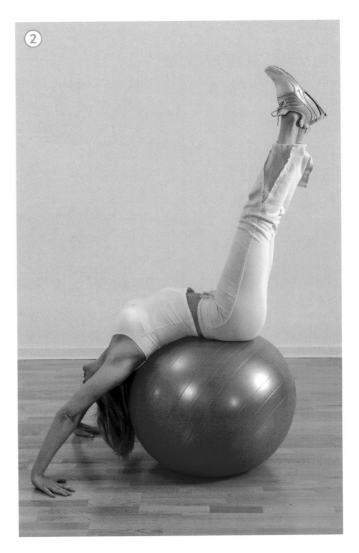

76

Oblique Cross to Knee

BENEFITS: Strengthens your oblique muscles and creates a curve in your waist.

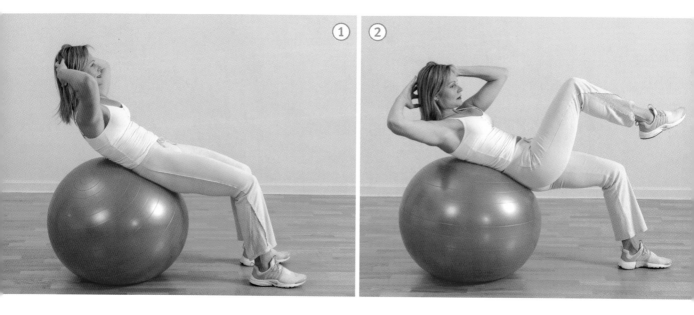

① ②

① Sit on the ball, just to the front of the top of the ball. Lie back into an incline position, with your hands behind your head.

② Lift one knee to the opposite elbow, pressing your trunk into the ball.

③ Return to the starting position and repeat on the other side. Do this 5 to 10 times on each side.

When holding your head in your hands, interlace your fingers, then drop your head into your hands, making sure that the hands are carrying the weight of the head—that's why they're placed there!

77

ADVANCED

Full Range Criss-Cross

BENEFITS: Further strengthens your oblique and transverse abdominal muscles.

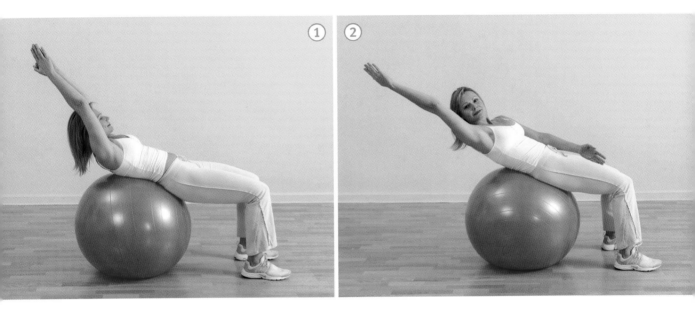

1. Lie over the ball on your back with your arms reaching behind your head.

2. As you sit up, reach one straight arm for the opposite knee, stretching the other arm out straight overhead.

3. Repeat 5 times on each side.

78 Incline Ab Crunches with Arms Straight Overhead

BENEFITS: Strengthens your rectus abdominal muscle without putting strain on your back.

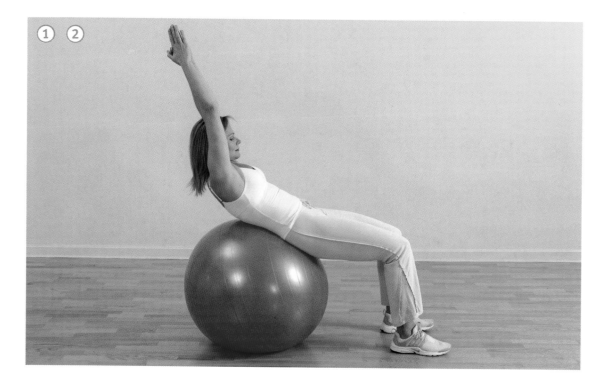

① Lie on your back on the ball in an incline. Reach your arms straight above your head with your elbows next to your ears and your hands clasped.

② Curl up, keeping your shoulders lowered and abs engaged.

③ Release and relax your back. Do this 8 to 10 times. You can do a second set if you want.

79

Wood Chop

BENEFITS: Strengthens your back and abdominal muscles, creating a long, lean torso.

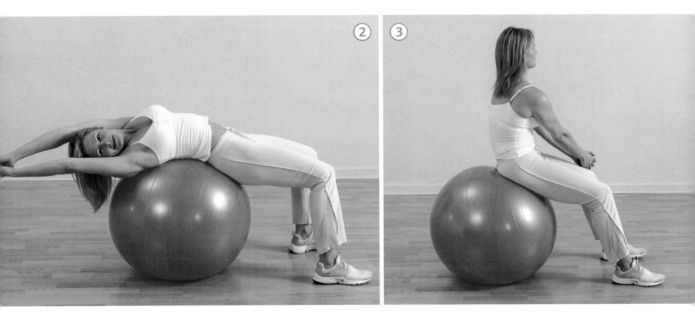

(1) Lie on your back on the ball, with your arms extended straight behind you, hands clasped.

(2) Reach both arms back into a long diagonal stretch, twisting to one side, keeping your hips evenly rooted into the ball.

(3) Roll up, bringing both arms up and over to the opposite thigh with a wood chopping action. Repeat 6 times on that side, then switch and do 6 to the other side.

80

Backstroke Abs

BENEFITS: Stretches your back, shoulders, and abdominal muscles while strengthening your stabilizing muscles.

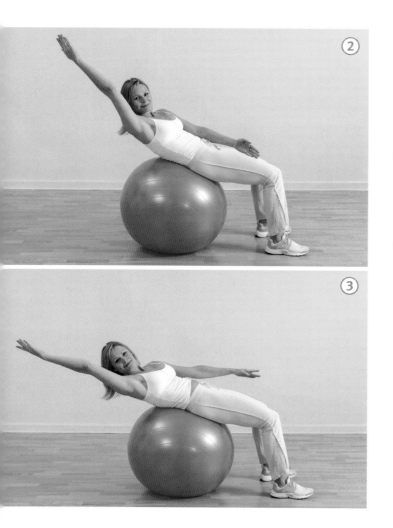

1. Lie on your back on the ball in a slightly inclined position. Your knees should be in line with your hips, your arms reaching forward in the scoop position.

2. Reach one straight arm back as the other arm stretches forward. Glance back at your hand, while your pelvis stays glued to the ball.

3. Circle your arm around, then change arms. Do this 4 times on each side.

81

Decline Abs Rolls

BENEFITS: Defines your rectus abdominal muscles.

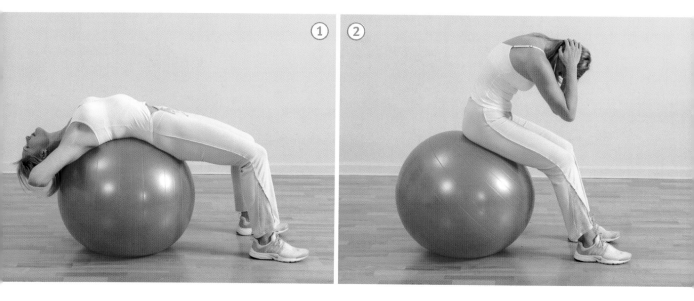

(1) Lie on your back over the ball with your rib cage past the top of the ball (towards the floor) and your hands behind your head, knees hip-distance apart. You can modify this exercise by lying more on top of the ball.

(2) Narrow your elbows and lift up into a crunch position in one count.

(3) Return slowly in 3 counts. Do this 8-10 times. You can do another set if you wish.

To increase the challenge, you can add a 2- to 4-pound medicine ball to this exercise. Hold it behind the middle of your skull, keeping your neck properly aligned.

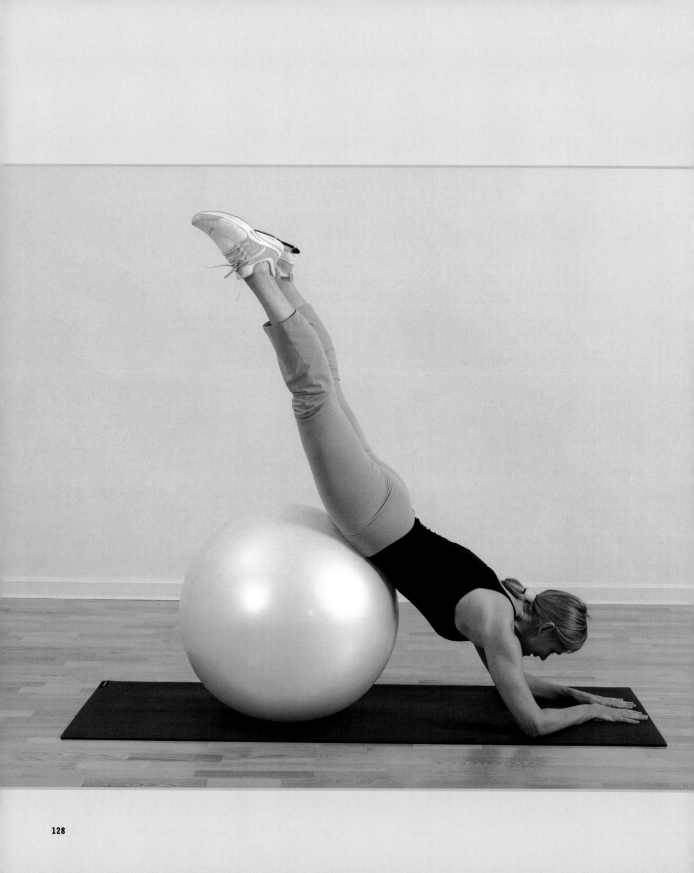

Prone Moves
on the Ball

People usually love to lie face down on the ball—it seems relaxing and they assume they won't have to work that hard. Oh, how wrong they are! Just because you're lying on your stomach doesn't mean you can't really work your muscles: Think about push-ups—you're not technically lying down, but you are face-down, and that's a killer move!

The prone position allows you to strengthen the back of your body—the muscles in your back and along your spine, as well as the backs of your legs. The muscles of your back include the trapezius (just below your neck), the rhomboids (below your shoulder blades), the latissumus dorsi (the sides of your back) and the erector spinae (the small muscles that run along your spinal column). If you're someone who sits at a desk all day, your back muscles are probably stretched forward and weak. If you lift heavy objects, or kids, you probably have imbalances in your back muscles. Most of us pick up and hold kids using one side of our body more than the other.

The following exercises will strengthen and stretch your back and leg muscles, allowing you to feel and look stronger as you go about your daily routine. The goal of most of these exercisers isn't to continually lift heavier and heavier weights. Most of us simply want to be able to look as good as we can and feel as strong and fit as possible. These exercises won't require you to lift lots of weights. Focus on your form and you'll notice improvement in your ability to move with control.

82 Bent Knee Upper Back Extension, Hands On Ball

BENEFITS: Strengthens the muscles of your middle back as well as those that run along your spinal column. Eases tension in your lower back.

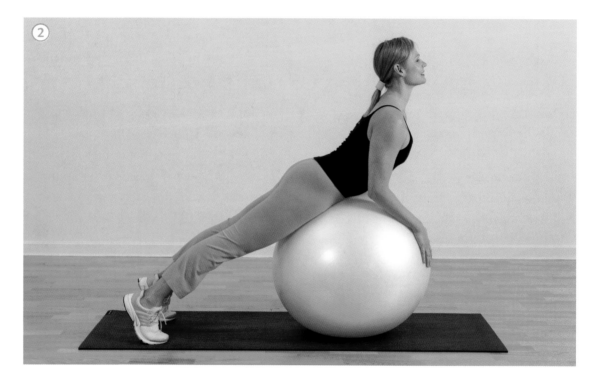

① Lie with your chest and pelvis over the ball, legs straight and hip-distance apart, balls of your feet planted firmly into the floor, and your hands on the ball in front of your chest.

② Pull the ball into your pelvis and extend your upper back, lifting your chest off the ball. Lower back to start. Repeat up to 8 times.

83

Prone Upper Back T-Pull

BENEFIT: Strengthens and stretches your rhomboids and trapezius muscles.

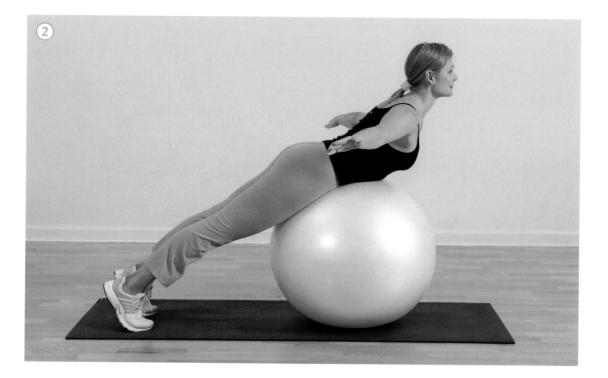

(1) Lie over the ball, knees slightly bent but off the floor, with arms in the T-position at shoulder-level, and neck long.

(2) Roll the ball forward straightening your legs as your arms lift and pull back towards your hips.

(3) Return to the starting position, and repeat 10 times.

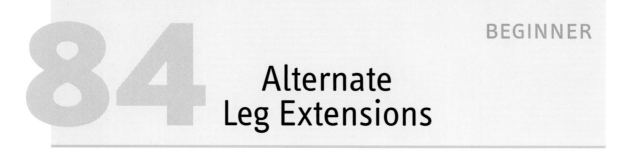

84 Alternate Leg Extensions

BENEFITS: Strengthens your hamstring and gluteus muscles; creates definition between your leg and butt.

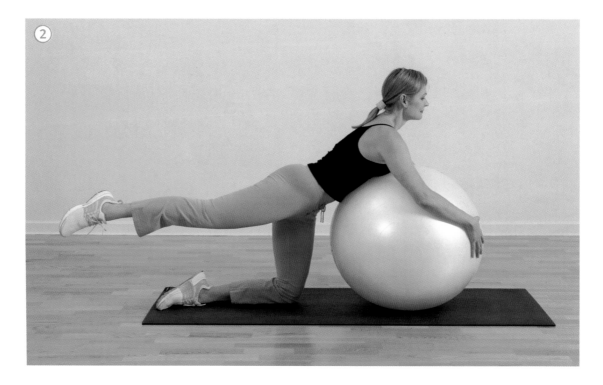

① Lie over the ball with your knees bent on the floor; pull the ball into your chest with your arms.

② Straighten one leg out from the bent position, then lift it off the floor to hip-height.

③ Return to the starting position and repeat with the other leg. Do this 10 times on each side.

85

Prone Straight Leg Lift with Push-Up

BENEFITS: Strengthens your chest, back, triceps, glutes, and hamstrings.

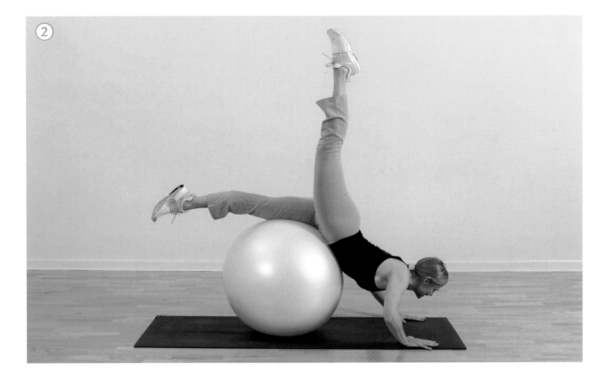

① Roll over the ball through prone position and into push-up position.

② Lift one leg off the ball, keeping both hip bones on the ball.

③ Roll the ball forward, bend your elbows, and bring your torso down.

④ Roll the ball back under your lower legs and repeat with the other leg. Work your way up to doing 10 on each side.

86 Two Leg Extension

BENEFITS: Strengthens the lower back and the muscles that run along the spine.

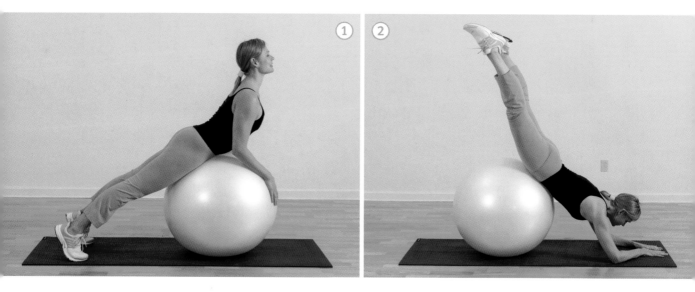

① Lie on the ball and roll forward to lean on your elbows, forearms, and hands.

② With your legs extended, roll forward, supporting yourself with your elbows on the floor, and lifting from your hips. Feel the contraction in your butt. Lower and repeat 5 times.

87

Prone Scissors

BENEFITS: Creates definition between your butt and your hamstrings.

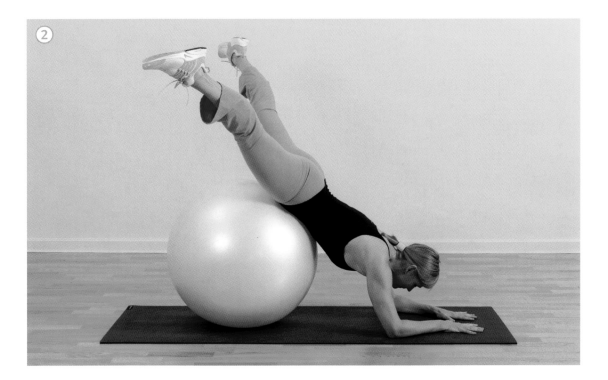

① Lie prone over the ball, your pelvis resting on the top of the ball, supporting yourself with your elbows. Be sure to line up your shoulders and wrists.

② Slowly open and close your legs in a wide scissors motion. Be sure to keep your spine in neutral and your abs engaged. When you're done, round your back like a hissing cat to stretch and reverse the curve of your spine. Repeat 5 times on each side.

88 Prone Double Hamstring Curl

BENEFITS: Lifts your butt.

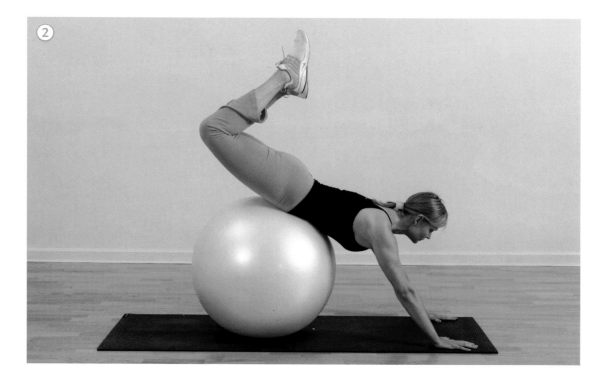

(1) Lie prone over the ball and roll forward, resting your hands on the floor to stabilize your shoulders. Be sure to keep your neck and shoulders relaxed and stretched away from each other. Your hips and thighs should be on top of the ball.

(2) Lift both knees off the ball, squeezing your butt and hamstrings away from the ball. Hold.

(3) Release both knees back to the ball. Repeat 5 times, working your way up to 10 times.

89 Prone Shoulder Roll

BENEFITS: Stretches the shoulder.

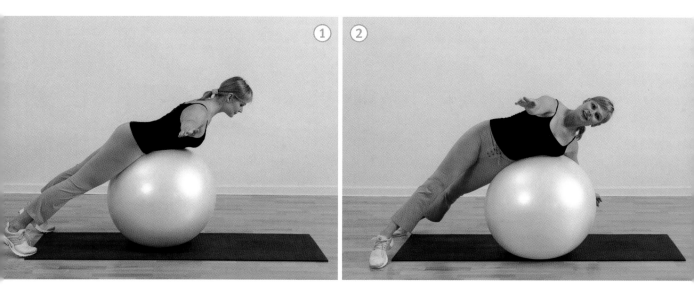

① Lie prone over the ball, and extend your legs straight out behind you, hip-distance apart. Keep your arms at shoulder height or a bit lower to keep your neck long and relaxed.

② Roll the ball towards one arm, turning onto your side while your arms stay in the lifted position.

③ Return to prone position. Repeat 5 times on each side.

90 Alternating Straight Leg Extensions

BENEFITS: Creates a lift in the butt. Strengthens the arms, back, shoulders, and abs.

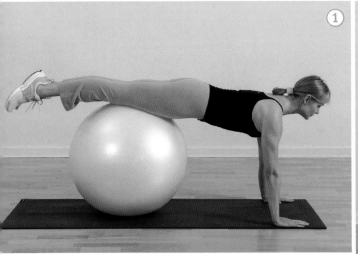

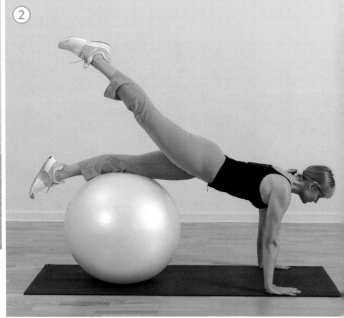

① ② Lie over the ball with a straight body—knees and shins on top of the ball and your hands on the floor in a push-up position.

② Keeping your hips perfectly even, lift one straight leg off the ball.

③ Return and repeat with your other leg. Repeat 10 times.

Grasshopper

BENEFITS: Isolates and strengthens your hamstrings, creating a curve in your back thigh.

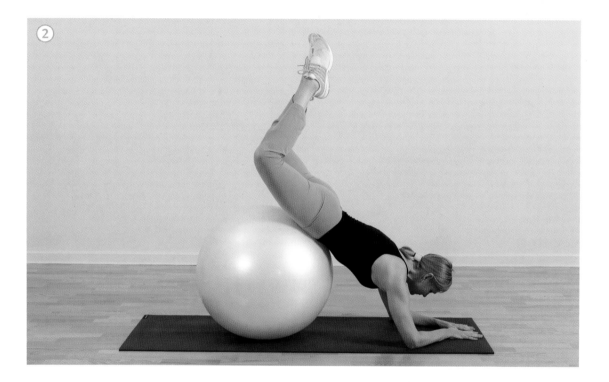

① Lie over the ball in a prone position with your upper thighs slightly turned out on the ball, your feet together and knees pointed out in a slight V, with your elbows on the floor.

② Lift both knees off the ball, while squeezing your butt. Do not tilt your pelvis or raise your back. Hold.

③ Return your knees to the ball. Repeat 5 times, working your way up to 10 times.

92 Swimming

BENEFITS: Strengthens the back muscles and shoulders.

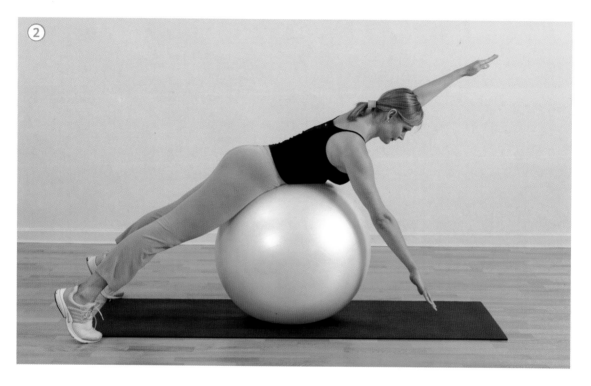

① Lie prone over the ball with your legs straight, hip-distance apart. Your full trunk should be on the ball and your arms straight at your sides.

② Pull your shoulder blades down, and away from your ears. Extend one arm—palm facing down—overhead, keeping your neck long.

③ Switch arms, extending out through your fingers and keeping your shoulders down the whole time. Repeat 5 times, working your way up to 10 times.

93

Push-Ups on the Ball at Knee Level

BENEFITS: Strengthens your upper body, especially your chest and back, and flattens your abs and core muscles.

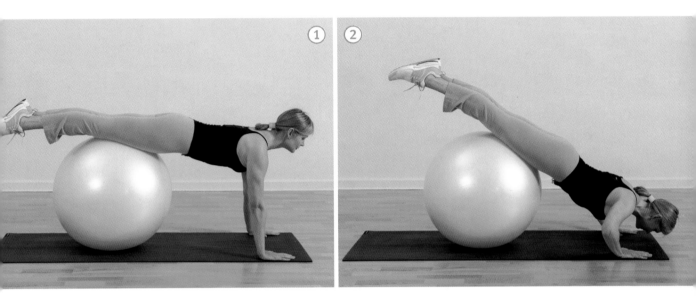

① Lie prone on the ball, then roll forward until your pelvis is off the ball and your knees are on top of the ball, arms supporting you in a push-up position. Stretch your body long in a straight plank. Your arms and hands should be directly under your shoulders, and your scapulae (shoulder blades) should be open and stable.

② Bend your elbows wide to your side, and make sure your chest lowers to the ground before your head. Repeat up to 8 times.

94 Push-Ups on Toes

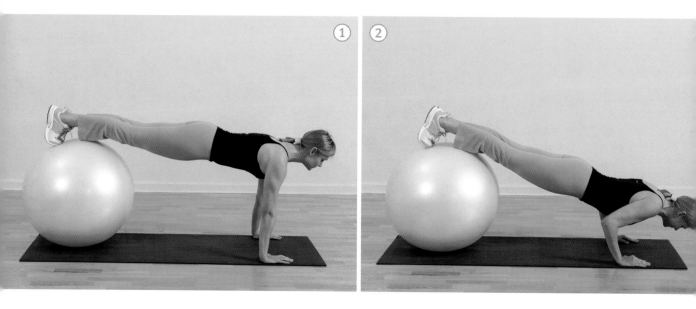

① Lie prone on the ball and roll out until your pelvis and thighs are off the ball and your toes are on top. Curl your toes under and stretch into a full push-up position, hands directly under your shoulders.

② Bend your elbows wide, keeping your body straight and the ball still, then straighten.

③ Hop feet off ball to finish. Repeat 2 to 10 times.

Yoga and Pilates
on the Ball

Yoga and Pilates are already great exercise systems on their own and, as I've said about Pilates, neither of them were created with the ball in mind. However, even the most dedicated and experienced yogi will find these new moves on the ball fun and challenging.

Both yoga and Pilates are considered mind/body systems because their goal is not to simply improve the look of your body, but also to fine-tune the way you relate to your body. And, in the case of yoga, the way you relate to your spirit and the way your spirit relates to the Universe.

Yoga and Pilates improve your mind/body connection by a) asking you to focus on your breath while you move and b) requiring you to move with your body and be in touch with the way your body feels, rather than simply, say, lifting ten pounds ten times in a row.

I've written a lot about Pilates in my introduction, but I want to take a minute or two to discuss yoga with you. The point of yoga is not to develop strong, lean bodies, although that is an added bonus! The point is to reach spiritual enlightenment. I can't actually promise that you'll do that with this workout—in fact, I can pretty much guarantee that you won't—but I can promise that if you do each of these moves with some breath awareness and a sense of calmness, you will experience both a relaxed body and a relaxed mind.

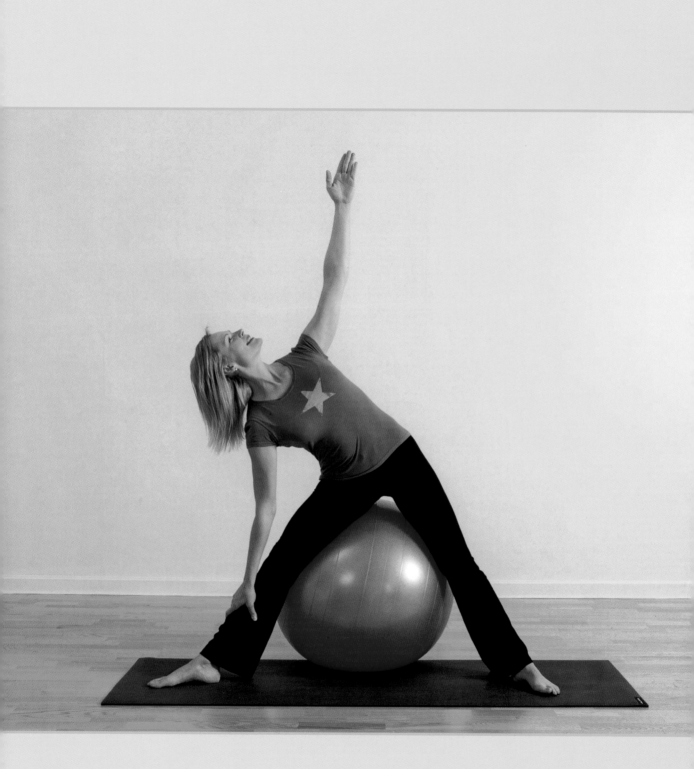

When doing a yoga exercise, focus on your breath, keeping the inhale and exhale long and slow. The reason so many people become yoga devotees is that they find a place within themselves that is calm and happy even while they are exercising or getting into a difficult position. So, if you notice that your body feels uncomfortable while you're in one of these postures, do what you can do make yourself more comfortable, take a deep breath, and try to consciously relax so that you don't even notice the position your body is in. How will this bring you to enlightenment? Well, if you can remain calm and centered while the world is swirling around you (or your body is in a funky pose) then you have a reached a higher level of consciousness.

But if you can't, don't worry! Remember, there is no judgment in yoga. It doesn't matter what you look like or what position your body ends up in. What's important is that your breath is calm and that your mind is rested. If you find yourself getting tense, try to relax more than trying to fix your body.

95 Oblique Saw on Ball

BENEFITS: The saw strengthens your lower back muscles and improves your posture. The spinal twist is also a great relief to sore backs.

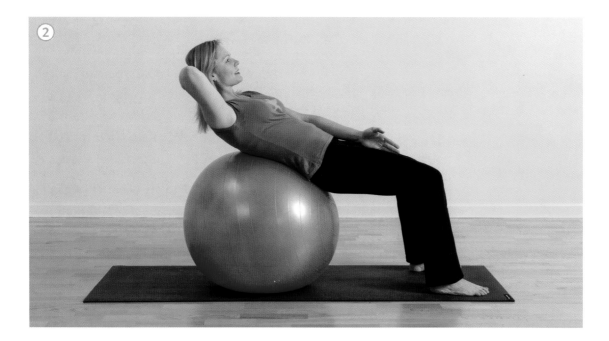

(1) Lie on your back on the ball, slightly inclined, with your knees and hips aligned, one hand behind your head. Cross one arm and hand to the outside of the opposite leg.

(2) Slide your hand—initiating very specifically from your arm, not your waist—up the outside of your thigh,

keeping your hips even and your rib cage pulling in opposition away from the motion of your arm. Lean forward with your whole torso.

(3) Return back to the starting position.

(4) Change to your other arm. Do 2 times on each side, working your way up to 5 times.

96

Teaser on Floor

BENEFITS: Improves your posture and the strength of your powerhouse muscles.

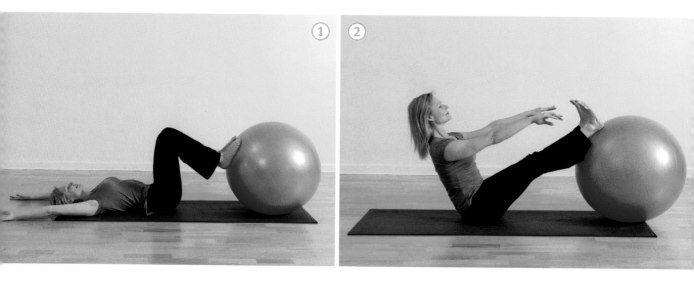

(1) Lie on your back with your heels on the ball, arms extended overhead, and knees bent.

(2) Roll the ball out as you straighten your legs and come to a sitting position, keeping your abs contracted, back long, and shoulders down.

97

Yoga Cat Stretch

BENEFITS: Totally relaxes your back and abs, as well as your neck and upper thighs.

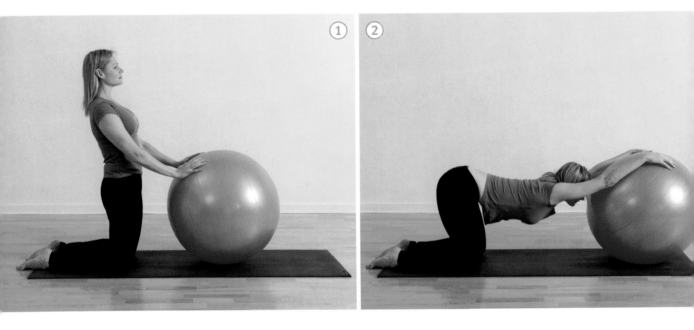

① Kneel on the floor, the ball in front of you, hands on top of the ball.

② Roll the ball forward, extending your spine into an arch.

Yoga Cat Stretch

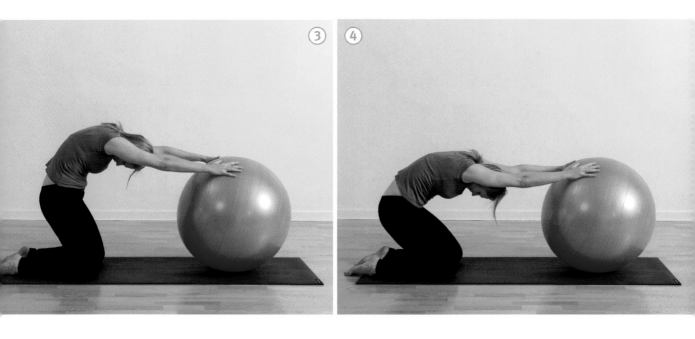

③ Roll the ball back, rounding your spine.

④ Roll back to the starting position, then lean back to stretch. You can do this as many times as you want!

98 Pike Handstand

BENEFITS: Strengthens all muscles of the body.

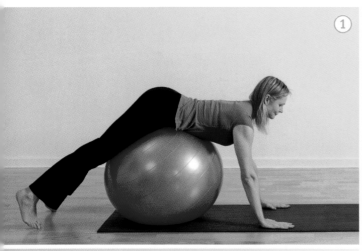

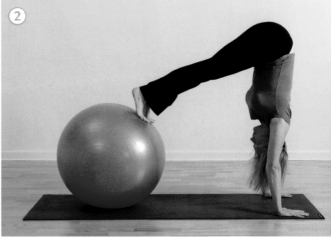

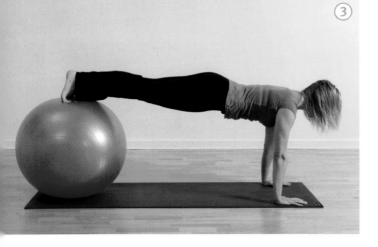

① Roll out to the push-up position.

② Roll the ball away with straight legs until your back is perpendicular and your toes are on top of the ball.

③ Reverse back to a push-up position. Do 1 time, working your way up to 3 or 5 times.

99

Yoga
Shoulder Stand

BENEFITS: Strengthens your upper body muscles, relaxes your legs and neck. Great for relieving tension.

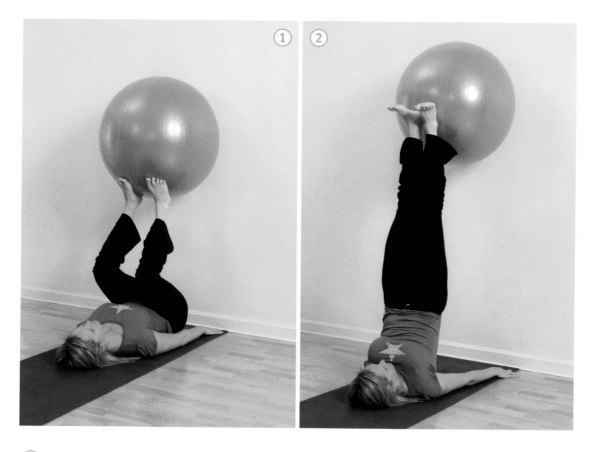

(1) Place the ball against a wall and support it with your feet, knees bent.

(2) Roll the ball up the wall into shoulder stand, using the ball as a support.

(3) Return to the starting position, rolling the ball down the wall. Do 1 time, or no more than 2 times.

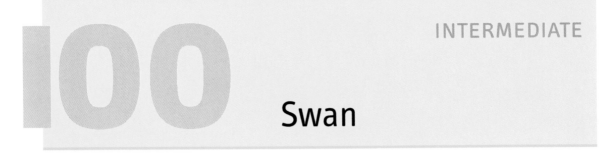 Swan

BENEFITS: A great exercise for strengthening your powerhouse and for shaping your torso and hips.

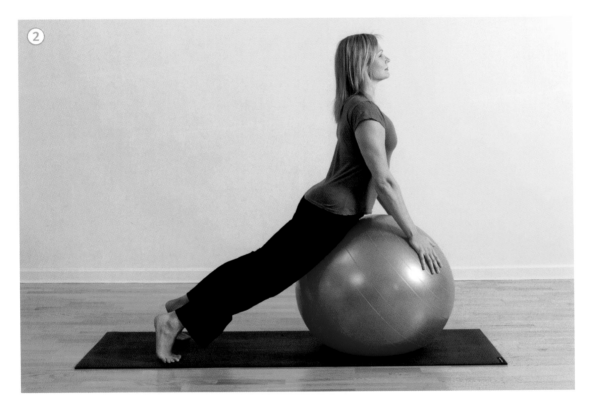

① Lie with your torso on the ball with arms down, and legs straight.

② Using your core muscles, inhale, and extend your head, neck, and shoulders up and away from the ball. Do not compress your lower spine by bending back too much.

③ Return and repeat 5 times.

101

Seated V-Sit
on the Ball

BENEFITS: One of the most difficult moves to achieve on the ball. When you can achieve this position, you'll know that you've really developed the strongest powerhouse possible.

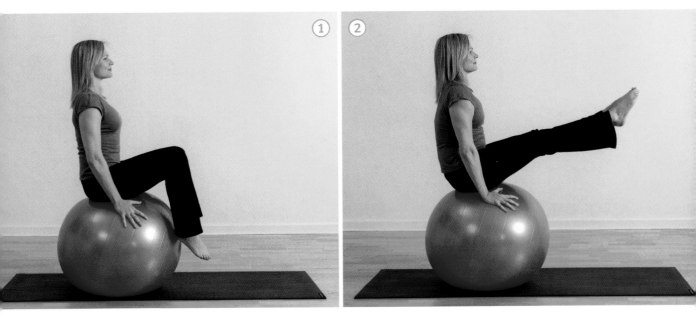

1. Sit on the ball with your hands on the ball by your hips, knees bent, feet on the ball.

2. Slowly extend your legs out straight into a V position. Hold and balance.

3. Return feet to the floor. Do 1 time and no more than 2 times.

102 BONUS MOVE
Cat Balance

BENEFITS: Makes you laugh!

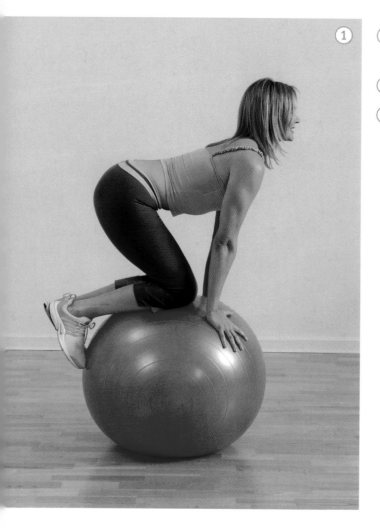

(1) Mount the top of the ball on all fours in a cat position.

(2) Balance.

(3) Fall off!! Ha ha. Once is enough!

Although I wrote this set of instructions with a sense of humor, I do feel it's my duty to tell you that there are more than a few of us dancers, athletes, and trainers who can not only balance on the ball, but who also perform a fair number of exercises in this precarious position. I've seen soccer players and other sports professionals practice catching medicine balls from all directions while balanced on the ball. So, while this pose may seem out of reach and a little silly, it's not! It's an example of what true core strength looks like, because someone whose powerhouse muscles are this strong really has total control of her body—and that was exactly what Joseph Pilates was looking for.

Creating Your Own Workouts

CHAPTER 10

The secret to creating an effective workout program is to know two things: 1) your goals and 2) how to reach them. (Actually, now that I think about it, that's actually the secret to success, too!) Anyway, I've created ten programs to get you started, but if you have another goal that I haven't listed, here are some tips on creating your own program.

1. Figure out what you want to achieve. For example, do you want to find a routine you can do in just fifteen minutes that will work your entire body? Or, are you looking to reach a certain physical goal, such as weight-loss?

2. Now, look through the book and read the benefits of each exercise. Write down the numbers of the exercises that look like they will help you reach your goals.

3. Think about which moves would work as a warm-up (easy moves that eventually get harder), and then a cool-down (moves that go from hard to easy), and then a logical sequence in the middle. You might want to work from standing to sitting to lying on the ball. Or, from one body part to another. Or, for a tougher workout, exhaust one body part by doing two or more exercises for it in a row.

4. Don't just stick with first program you create. Changes in your body only happen when the muscles are continually surprised, so try your sequences for a week or two and then create a new routine. You might want to do the moves in reverse or just pick new moves for the same muscle groups. Once that two-week period is up, you can go back to your first routine. You'll find that your body adapts to the exercises over time, so that when you come back to ones you did before, you can do them with better form and more control.

Complete 15-Minute Core Workout

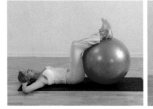 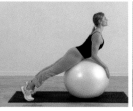 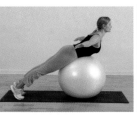 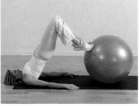

55   **Floor Criss-Cross**
(page 98)

82   **Bent Knee Upper Back Extension**
(page 130)

83   **Prone Upper Back T-Pull**
(page 131)

74   **Pelvic Lifts**
(page 120)

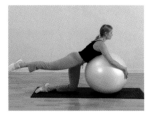

84   **Alternate Leg Extensions**
(page 132)

15-Minute Morning Wake-Up

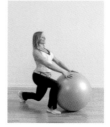

9 Standing Lateral
Side Bend
(page 43)

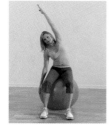

28 Seated Side Lifts
(page 64)

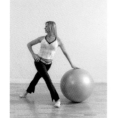

100 Swan
(page 152)

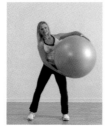

11 Figure 8
(page 45)

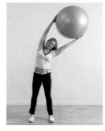

12 Rolling Front Lunge
(page 46)

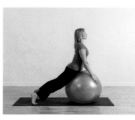

14 Twisting Spiral
Lunge, Hand on Hip
(page 48)

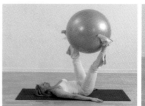

66 Inner Thigh Twists
(page 111)

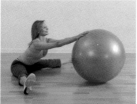

34 Seated Forward Roll
(page 70)

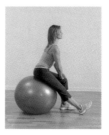

31 Seated Hamstring
Stretch
(page 67)

Total Body Strengthening

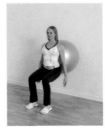

16   **Ball Wall Squats**
(page 50)

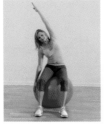

28   **Seated Side Bends**
(page 64)

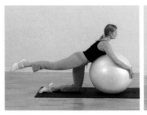

84   **Alternate Leg
Extensions**
(page 132)

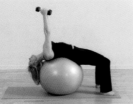

53   **Decline Chest Flies**
(page 93)

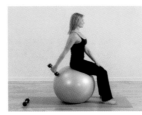

48   **Seated Tricep Taps**
(page 88)

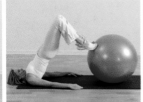
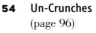

61   **Supine Pelvic
Press Up**
(page 106)

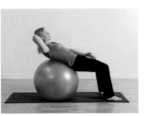

54   **Un-Crunches**
(page 96)

95   **Oblique Saw on Ball**
(page 146)

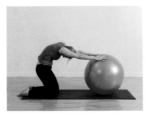

97   **Yoga Cat Stretch**
(page 148)

Agility Workout

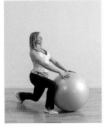

12 Rolling Front Lunge
(page 46)

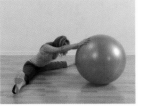

35 Extended Forward
Roll
(page 71)

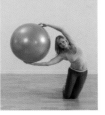

32 Kneeling Side Bend
Stretch
(page 68)

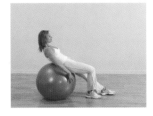

60 Walking Spinal Roll
(page 105)

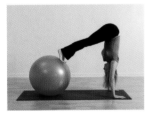

98 Pike Handstand
(page 150)

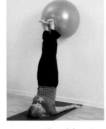

75 Backbend Balance
(page 121)

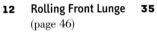

99 Yoga Shoulder Stand
(page 151)

Core Workout

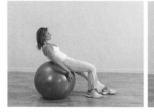

60 **Walking Spinal Roll**
(page 105)

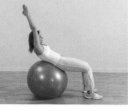

78 **Incline Ab Crunches with Arms Straight Overhead**
(page 124)

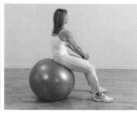

79 **Wood Chop**
(page 125)

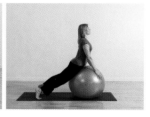

100 **Swan**
(page 152)

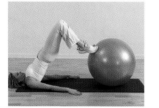

69 **Rolling Bridge on Toes**
(page 115)

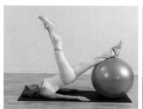

63 **Diamond Hip Lifts**
(page 108)

64 **Supine Alternate Straight Leg Lifts**
(page 109)

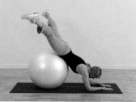

87 **Prone Scissors**
(page 135)

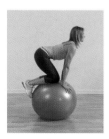

102 **Cat Balance**
(page 154)

15-Minute Ab Strengthener

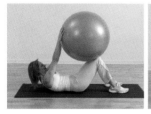

54 "Un-Crunches" (page 96)

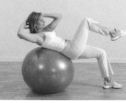

76 Oblique Cross to Knee (page 122)

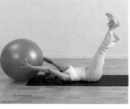

56 Reverse Crunch on Floor (page 100)

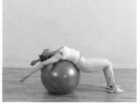

72 Uncrunches on the Ball (page 118)

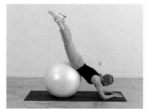

86 Two Leg Extension (page 134)

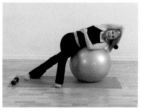

84 Alternate Leg Extensions (page 132)

91 Grasshopper (page 139)

51 Side Bends with Weight and Straight Leg (page 91)

30-Minute
Total Body Toner

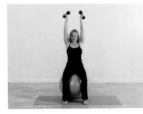

37   3-D Shoulder Press
(page 76)

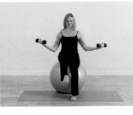

40   Seated Bicep Curls
with Single Leg Lift
(page 80)

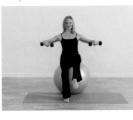

50   Lateral Shoulder
Raises, One Leg
Raised
(page 90)

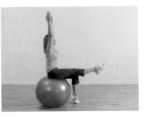

36   Leg Extensions
(page 72)

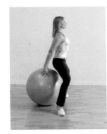

17   2nd Position
Grande Plié
(page 51)

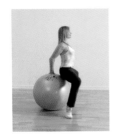

23   2nd Position with
Tricep Dips
(page 57)

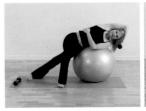

51   Side Bends with
Weight and
Straight Leg
(page 91)

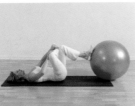

73   Ball Hip Rotator
Stretch
(page 119)

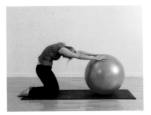

97   Yoga Cat Stretch
(page 148)

Total Body Workout

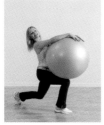 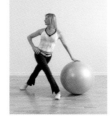 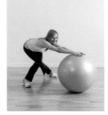 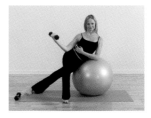

19 Perfect Lunges: Front Ball Hug (page 53)

14 Twisting Spiral Lunge, Hand on Hip (page 48)

24 Full Twisting Two-Handed Spiral Lunge (page 58)

47 Side Bend on Ball with Weights (page 87)

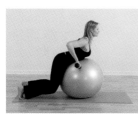 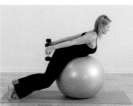 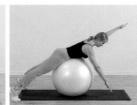 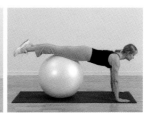

49 Prone Upper Back Rows (page 89)

52 Prone Tricep Extensions (page 92)

92 Swimming (page 140)

93 Push-Ups on the Ball at Knee Level (page 141)

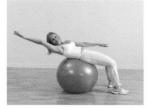 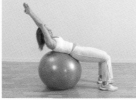 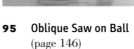

80 Backstroke Abs (page 126)

77 Full-Range Criss-Cross (page 123)

95 Oblique Saw on Ball (page 146)

10-Minute Energizer

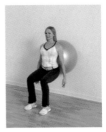

16   Ball Wall Squats
(page 50)

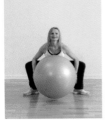

20   Frog Jumps
(page 54)

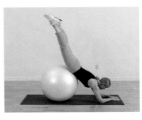

86   Two Leg Extension
(page 134)

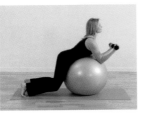

43   Decline Bicep Curls
over Ball
(page 83)

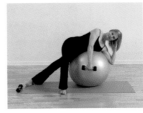

44   Side Lying Fly
(page 84)

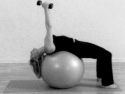

45   Decline Bench Press
(page 85)

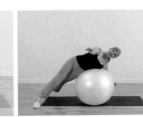

46   Overhead Triceps
Press
(page 86)

89   Prone Shoulder Roll
(page 137)

Total Body Tone

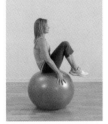

30 Seated Knee
Crunches
(page 66)

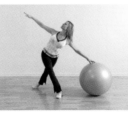

96 Teaser on Floor
(page 147)

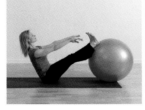

15 Extended Spiral
Lunge
(page 49)

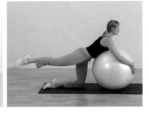

84 Alternate Leg
Extensions
(page 132)

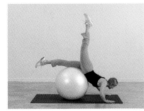

85 Prone Straight Leg
Lift with Push-Up
(page 133)

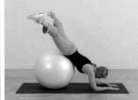

87 Prone Scissors
(page 135)

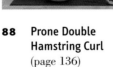

88 Prone Double
Hamstring Curl
(page 136)

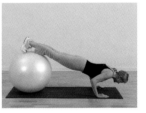

94 Push-Ups on Toes
(page 142)

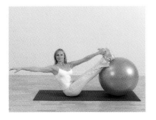

57 Teaser with Twist
(page 102)

15-Minute Leg Lengthener

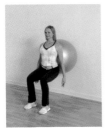

16 **Ball Wall Squats**
(page 50)

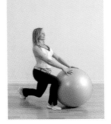

12 **Rolling Front Lunge**
(page 46)

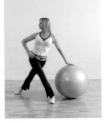

14 **Twisting Spiral Lunge, Hand on Hip**
(page 48)

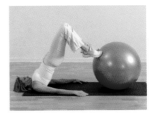

74 **Pelvic Lifts**
(page 120)

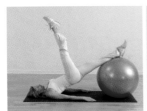

64 **Supine Alternate Straight Leg Lifts**
(page 109)

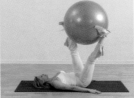

66 **Inner Thigh Twists**
(page 111)

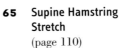

65 **Supine Hamstring Stretch**
(page 110)

15-Minute Butt Blaster

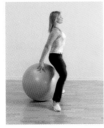

17 2nd Position Grande Plié
(page 51)

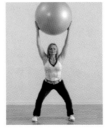

18 Squats
(page 52)

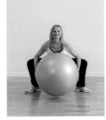

20 Frog Jumps
(page 54)

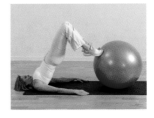

74 Pelvic Lifts
(page 120)

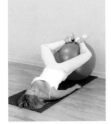

63 Diamond Hip Lifts
(page 108)

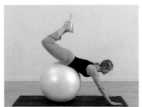

88 Prone Double Hamstring Curl
(page 136)

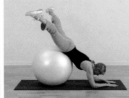

87 Prone Scissors
(page 135)

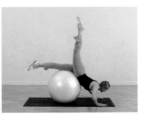

85 Prone Straight Leg Lift with Push-Up
(page 133)

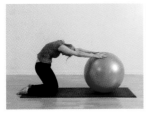

97 Yoga Cat Stretch
(page 148)

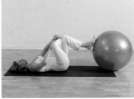

73 Ball Hip Rotator Stretch
(page 119)

15-Minute
Back Strengthener

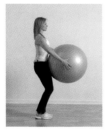

8   **Standing Lat Stretch**
(page 42)

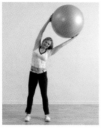

9   **Standing Lateral Side Bend**
(page 43)

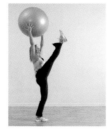

22   **Standing Front Leg Lifts**
(page 56)

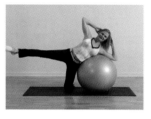

25   **Side Bend with Straight Leg Side Lift**
(page 59)

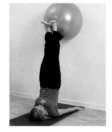

99   **Yoga Shoulder Stand**
(page 151)

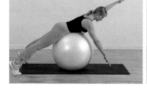

92   **Swimming**
(page 140)

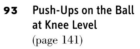

93   **Push-Ups on the Ball at Knee Level**
(page 141)

15-Minute Arm Toner

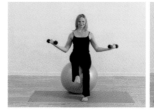

40 Seated Bicep Curls
with Single Leg Lift
(page 80)

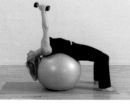

53 Decline Chest Press
(page 93)

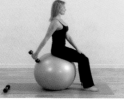

48 Seated Tricep Taps
(page 88)

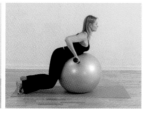

49 Prone Upper Back
Rows
(page 89)

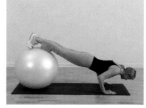

94 Push-Ups on Toes
(page 142)

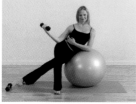

47 Side Bend on Ball
with Weights
(page 87)

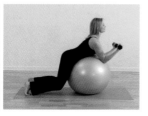

37 3-D Shoulder Press
(page 76)

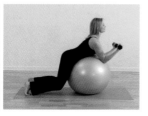

43 Decline Bicep Curls
over Ball
(page 83)

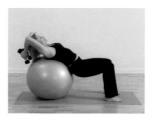

46 Overhead Triceps
Press
(page 86)

15-Minute Relaxation

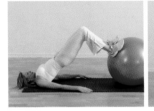

62 Hamstring Roll
(page 107)

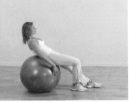

60 Walking Spinal Roll
(page 105)

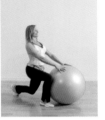

12 Rolling Front Lunge
(page 46)

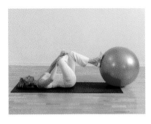

73 Ball Hip Rotator
Stretch
(page 119)

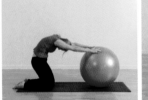

97 Yoga Cat Stretch
(page 148)

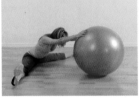

35 Extended Forward
Roll
(page 71)

15-Minute
Bedtime Soother

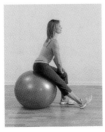

31 Seated Hamstring
Stretch
(page 67)

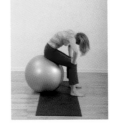

6 Full Spinal Flexion
(page 39)

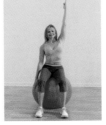

5 Single Sliding Arm
Side Stretch
(page 38)

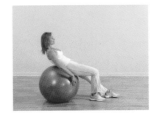

60 Walking Spinal Roll
(page 105)

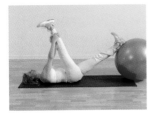

65 Supine Hamstring
Stretch
(page 110)

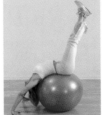

75 Backbend Balance
(page 121)

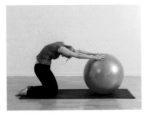

97 Yoga Cat Stretch
(page 148)

Ball Glossary

Apex: the very top of the ball

Core: The muscles of your trunk, including your spine, upper back, lower back, chest, and abdominals. Also called the powerhouse.

Decline: Lying with your feet higher than your hips, or your hips higher than your head.

Hip distance: When I say, "place your feet hip-distance apart," I mean situating your feet directly under your hip bones.

Incline: Lying with your head higher than your hips, or your hips higher than your feet.

Neutral spine: Your lower back should not be tilted forward or swayed back.

Neutral pelvis: Your pelvis should be relaxed, not contracted or swaying back.

Powerhouse: The muscles of your trunk, including your spine, upper back, lower back, chest, and abdominals.

Prone: Lying face-down, on the ball or on the floor.

Pulse: Similar to a gentle bounce, you can pulse your body as you stretch without forcing any movement.

Scapula retraction: Pulling shoulder blades down, away from your ears.

Supine: Lying face up, either on the ball or on the floor.

Tripod of the pelvis: Sitting in such a way so that the front of your pelvis and your sitting bones are equally weighted on the ball or on the floor. You're not leaning forward or back.

Acknowledgments

Writing this book has been THE most challenging and gratifying accomplishment so far in my twenty-year professional career.

A huge hug and thank you to Holly Schmidt, for believing in my expertise and selecting me for this project. Her reassurance and support got me through the hurdles of writing my first book! You're an amazing publisher.

Thank you to the helpful staff at Fair Winds, and Rockport Publishers, especially Silke Braun and Claire MacMaster. I appreciate their great art direction and hospitality—making sure I arrived on time for days of photo shoots, and helping to inflate those balls! Dalyn Miller, thanks for the fine dining and cross-promoting strategies.

Thanks to the staff at Hair Works in Gloucester, Mass., for making me look beautiful and to the amazing Allan Penn for my best photos yet! Bevan Walker, thanks for a great eye! Thanks also to Brigid Carroll and Rhiannon Soucy for their help with the manuscript.

For Donna Raskin, my editor, and a great person. A very special sincere thank you. You sequestered me for this project, and I am so appreciative. Thanks for hearing my voice, and guiding me through "the process" with patience and flexibility… let's do it again sometime! Now that my computer is fixed. Thanks to Hill Street Computers who opened for me on a Sunday to fix my computer and John came to the rescue ridding me of seven viruses. What an experience and period of growth for me.

A heartfelt thanks to all who support my out-of-the-box ideas and cover my work schedule, believing its important for me to be able to share my work on a larger scale.

Thank you to my teaching staff for your loyalty and for working with me for years at my Insidescoop Studios in NY. Charmain Surface, a.k.a. "boss lady," couldn't have done it all without you! Angelique Christensen my protégé extraordinaire who covers for my schedule in a moment's notice. Corey Carver and Meghan—generous teachers and assistants who keep me organized. Mom, thanks for never missing a day at the desk.

Thanks to Hollis Sloam, Vivian Legunn, Cornelia Guest, Helene Fortunoff, David Colburn, Monica Forman, Hina Tanner, Mila Kristy Kulsa—who recently skated for gold, proving my ball for hips successful—Caroline Kuperschmidt, and Shelly Haber. Their injuries, and their will to overcome, inspired me to design a lot of the exercises in this book.

Thank you to Andrea Ambandos, an un-paralleled producer for my consumer market video exposure, and caring enough to bring out the best in me. Thank you Mellissa McNeese for the best *Fit* PR exposure ever. Thanks to Koch Vision, especially Lucille Deane, for working on my new video line, and Angela Sorti for the new Web site design. Thanks to Michael Koch for believing in my name as a great new talent, and executive producing my tapes. Thank you to Michelle Rygiel at Anchor Bay for hiring me to write and star in the *Stability Ball for Dummies* workout. Howard Maier, thank you for the platform to test my talents as Pilates artistic director of Yoga Zone. A special thank you to my lawyer Van Cushny for his counsel. Thank you also to Al Amadio, my other attorney, whose kindness got me through a very tough time. Thank you Jacamo at Shishkabob for greeting me with hugs and hummus! On 4-hour work days my big fat Greek diet really works!

Finally, an unmeasurable thanks to my Mom, Glory Gillies, who has always made me believe I am special and expects the best from me and who is always there to run my studio and baby-sit. Thanks to my amazing daughter Cadence, the sunshine of my life, whose personality brightens up any room.

In closing, thanks to a special person, Dr. Geraldine Costa, whose positive influence continues to give me the strength to face my fears in my life's journey. Thanks for being my mentor in business, a best friend and fan, and nurturing my personal growth for twenty-one years. Thanks to her husband, Dr. Sydney Cohen, for taking my Pilates class and recognizing my talent when I was still in high school. You were my first private clients who made my success possible.

About the Author

Liz Gillies develops and stars in numerous videos including *Zone Pilates*, *Stability Ball Workouts*, *Stability Ball for Dummies*, and her own "Core Fitness" line of videos. She is the owner and artistic director of The Insidescoop Studios in New York, where she has been certifying teachers in the Pilates method since 1997. She has been featured in numerous news programs and national publications.

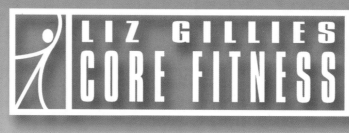

LIZ GILLIES CORE FITNESS

Completely Transform Your Body!

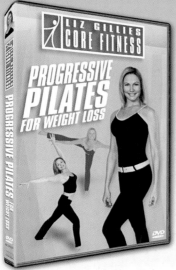

Learn Liz Gillies Core Fitness techniques to create long, lean muscles; strong, flat abs and a sleek silhouette without bulking up!

PROGRESSIVE PILATES FOR WEIGHT LOSS

Get in touch with your body's core and sculpt leaner legs and a firm butt. Kick your Pilates practice up a notch with this energetic workout that combines standing dance fundamentals with weight bearing movements. The traditional Pilates technique is transformed to a fat-burning pace that will enable you to burn more calories and give you dramatic results quickly.

Includes a bonus 10 minute Abs Blast!

Available on DVD and VHS!

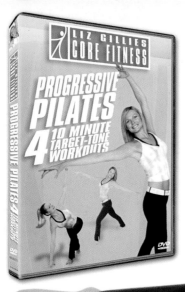

PROGRESSIVE PILATES — FOUR TEN-MINUTE TARGET-TONE WORKOUTS

Make every minute of your workout count by targeting your body's core! These four effective workouts focus on the abs, butt, arms and thighs. Liz's 3-dimensional approach to classic Pilates mat exercises will tone, firm and re-shape your body using focused concentration and precise form. You will improve muscle coordination, increase energy and improve your overall fitness.

Includes a bonus 10-minute Total Body Weight Loss Challenge!

Visit www.kochvision.com for news and updates!